Essential Elements of Wound Diagnosis

Rose Hamm, PT, DPT
Adjunct Assistant Professor of Clinical Physical Therapy
Division of Biokinesiology and Physical Therapy
University of Southern California
Los Angeles, California

Joseph N. Carey, MD
Plastic Surgery Program Director
Assistant Professor of Surgery
Assistant Professor of Neurological Surgery
University of Southern California
Keck School of Medicine
Los Angles, California

New York   Chicago   San Francisco   Athens   London   Madrid   Mexico City
Milan   New Delhi   Singapore   Sydney   Toronto

Essential Elements of Wound Diagnosis

1 2 3 4 5 6 7 8 9 DSS 26 25 24 23 22 21

ISBN 978-1-260-46047-6
MHID 1-260-46047-9

The editors were Michael Weitz and Christina M. Thomas
The production supervisor was Catherine Saggese.
The text designer was Mary McKeon.
Project management was provided by Rishabh Gupta, MPS Limited.

Library of Congress Cataloging-in-Publication Data

Names: Hamm, Rose, author. | Carey, Joseph, 1973- author.
Title: Essential elements of wound diagnosis / Rose Hamm, Joseph Carey.
Description: New York : McGraw Hill, [2021] | Includes bibliographical
   references and index. | Summary: "The evaluation of the patient with a
   non-healing wound consists of three components - subjective history,
   medical history, and wound assessment. The histories will usually allow
   the clinician to make a diagnosis of wound etiology, and if not, at
   least know what needs to be ruled out. They will also give indications
   as to why the wound is not healing. The wound assessment provides data
   for objective, measurable outcomes and progress, as well as information
   on how to treat the wound initially. The most important aspects of
   treating any wound are to treat all underlying co-morbidities and to
   address any issues that may be impeding wound healing. Finally, the
   initial treatment will consist of appropriate debridement of necrotic
   tissue and application of a dressing that will ensure adequate moisture
   for wound healing to advance"— Provided by publisher.
Identifiers: LCCN 2020029693 (print) | LCCN 2020029694 (ebook) | ISBN
   9781260460476 (paperback) | ISBN 9781260460469 (ebook)
Subjects: MESH: Wounds and Injuries—complications | Wounds and
   Injuries—therapy | Wound diagnosis | Wound Healing
Classification: LCC RD93 (print) | LCC RD93 (ebook) | NLM WO 700 | DDC
   617.1—dc23
LC record available at https://lccn.loc.gov/2020029693
LC ebook record available at https://lccn.loc.gov/2020029694

Dedication

The authors gratefully and respectfully
dedicate this book
to the many patients who have
entrusted us with their care, and who
in doing so, have taught us much of what
we know about diagnosing and treating patients
with non-healing wounds.

Contents

Reviewers

David G. Armstrong, DPM, MD, PhD
Professor of Surgery
Director, Southwestern Academic Limb
Salvage Alliance (SALSA)
Keck School of Medicine
University of Southern California
Los Angeles, California

Young Jin Kwak, MD, FAAD, FACMS
Mohs Micrographic Surgery and
Dermatologic Oncology
Laser Skin Care Specialists
Long Beach, California

Adam L. Isaac, DPM
Director of Research
Foot and Ankle Specialists of the
Mid-Atlantic
Rockville, Maryland

Preface

When the first edition of *Text and Atlas of Wound Diagnosis and Treatment* was published, a physician friend said to me, "If I have a patient with a wound in my office, and I don't know what it is, I do not have the time to go through this book and find it." From that conversation, the idea originated for a pictorial reference that practicing clinicians could use to diagnose unusual wounds, and thus have a starting point for developing a plan of care, including appropriate referrals to other medical specialists.

The mission of this work, in addition to aiding diagnosis, is to stress that every wound is on a patient, and it is the patient who is being treated first and foremost. Yes, the wound requires attention directly, but concurrently, patient concerns, conditions, and circumstances must be specifically addressed as well. These include co-morbidities, nutrition, complete system review, functional status, and personal habits, as well as social, psychological, and economic factors. An inter-disciplinary approach to treating patients with wounds is often required for the best outcomes; thus the information included in this book is intended to be applicable and useful for all of the medical professions.

The principles of evidence-based wound care are discussed in the first chapter as a guide to caring for any patient with a wound, including the recommended supplies needed for care during the first encounter. However, "clean, cut, and cover" as a treatment model does not constitute evidence-based wound care and often adjunct therapies such as compression therapy, biophysical agents, advanced dressings, nutritional counseling, exercise, or hyperbaric oxygen therapy are recommended to advance healing, prevent infection, and achieve faster closure. Therefore, the sections on medical management and wound management are intended to suggest to the primary caregiver referrals that may be beneficial in achieving faster healing, thus helping to prevent the risk of complications, saving cost of care, and improving patient satisfaction.

My goal as a clinician was to treat a wound in such a way that the patient did not have to provide care between treatment sessions; the patient's responsibility was to get on with life in as normal a way as possible. This was accomplished by performing appropriate debridement, using advanced dressings, and providing adequate patient education. Interestingly, much of this book was written during the COVID-19 pandemic of 2020. During this time, much of patient care was transitioned to telemedicine—i.e. teaching the patient or the caregiver how to manage the wound at home with less hands-on care by the clinician. This has allowed us to evaluate our previous methods and to compare them to a higher level of involvement of the patient and caregiver in the home setting. Time and research will hopefully reflect on the two different approaches and tell us which method produces the best outcomes. Regardless of how the patient and the wound are treated, an accurate diagnosis is the first very critical component of good care. To that end, we hope that you find the photographs and text beneficial in your practice.

The wounds covered in this book reflect the myriad of cases that we have seen in the combined thirty-plus years that we have practiced wound care. And each of you could add some from your own experiences, which we would welcome having you send to us so they can be included in the next edition. Students are often told that once they get into the clinic, the patients become their best teachers. We are incredibly grateful to all of those patients who have so graciously trusted us to provide their care and have taught us through their open honesty. God bless you as you work to care for His people who have chronic, non-healing, or atypical wounds; may you always be open to what those patients have to teach you.

Rose Hamm, DPT
Joseph Carey, MD

Foreword

Every person sustains injuries that can sometimes result in dermal wounds. These wounds almost always require active healing by the patient. Fortunately, millions of years of evolution have resulted in exquisitely sensitive, redundant, and effective healing mechanisms. While most of these wounds heal without clinician intervention, some do not. That is the focus of *Essential Elements of Wound Diagnosis* and why the information in this book is so important. For the physician, nurse, physical therapist or wound clinician, knowing the clues for problem wounds and having a scheme to treat them can be essential to a happy patient with a healing wound.

This book is based on the experiences of two busy clinicians who have worked together for years. It provides an organized approach to the diagnosis of wounds and their care. These are documented with great photographs that will help a treating clinician to recognize the problem their patient has presented and to begin a treatment that is practical and mechanistic. This is the kind of reference that every practice should have easily available. I hope the reader will appreciate the decades of experience and hundreds of patients who are in the background. This is a book to read, but then return to again and again.

Congratulations to the authors for a job well done!

Warren Garner, MD, FACS
Professor of Surgery
Keck School of Medicine, USC

Acknowledgements

Every completed book depends upon an editorial staff that is supportive, encouraging, and patient with the authors—the staff at McGraw Hill Education has been all of that and more. From the first verbalization of this book's concept, Michael Weitz has been awesome, always believing in the project and trusting our professional judgment about what to include and exclude. Making those judgments has not been an easy task, and Michael's belief in our choices has been invaluable to our confidence in making the right decisions. During the process of doing two books and 52 posts on AccessPhysiotherapy, Michael has been not only a treasured editor, but also a caring friend.

The editorial staff, headed by Christina Thomas, has been the epitome of patience and professionalism as she kept us on track and on time. With much of the book being written during the COVID-19 pandemic, being on schedule was at times challenging, especially for Dr. Carey as he juggled patient care, surgery, clinics, and family safety. We are deeply grateful to Christina for guiding us through this difficult time with such grace. The Permissions Co-ordinator, Sheryl Krato, did a fantastic job of ensuring that every photograph and figure was appropriately credited. Those kinds of details are definitely not the forte of authors, and we so appreciate her detail to credibility! The art department, including Anthony Landi, was creative in designing a cover that would be relative to the book's content, yet palatable to non-clinicians who might pick up a copy, although the authors are quick to inform friends that this is not a coffee table book! A very special thank you goes to Jeffrey Thompson, DPT, at Keck Hospital of USC, for providing the photograph for the cover. His photograph depicts the ideal set-up for providing an individual treatment using a sterile field and instruments, as discussed in Chapter 1. Our gratitude is also extended to Production Supervisor Catherine Saggese and Text Designer Mary McKeon. The first time I saw a pdf of the text with the chapter designs, I thought "Wow, this is pretty and eye-catching!" and as my grandchildren have heard me say many times, "Esthetics count." I hope you enjoy the beauty of the book as much as I do. MPS Limited, headed by Rishabh Gupta, did an awesome job of formatting the pages in such a way that the photographs and text coordinate in order to make the information easy for the reader to relate and assimilate. Thank you to everyone involved in making this dream idea a tangible reality!

Our sincere gratitude is extended to Dr. David Armstrong, Dr. Adam Isaac, and Dr. Young Kwak for their gracious reviews, valuable comments and suggestions, and professional expertise which they so willingly shared. There is no way the authors could be experts in every topic covered in this type of reference book, and having their experienced and knowledgeable review and critique of the content was very reassuring for us.

A huge thank you is extended to our colleagues at Keck Hospital for all they have shared with us over the years, adding to our knowledge base and stimulating us to learn more and be better clinicians. To paraphrase an old saying, no author is an island, and it takes many teachers, mentors, and colleagues to make one a successful provider of medical care. Our teachers and colleagues at the Keck School of Medicine, Keck Hospital, and the Division of Biokinesiology and Physical Therapy have been the best! Dr. Warren Garner, Director of the Burn Unit at LA County/USC Hospital has been a mentor for both authors, and we are especially honored that he was willing to write the Foreword.

Our families have been very understanding, supportive, and patient as we spend time at the computer, researching and writing, to make this concept a reality. Every reference, every topic, every sentence, and every word is critically selected to provide the reader with the most recent and accurate information in the most succinct way. The focus required in accomplishing the work often means missing questions and comments from loved ones, as well as missing precious time with them, and their support is irreplaceable.

Lastly, as is stated in the dedication, we thank all of the patients whom we have been privileged to care for during our professional careers. They are indeed our best teachers, most valued support group, and often become our dear friends. To be in the medical profession at any level is an honor beyond words, demanding trust that is indescribable, both between provider and patient and between colleagues. We have been blessed to work in a medical community at Keck Hospital that is the epitome of collegiality, and we hope that we are able to extend that sense of professional companionship and cooperation to all who are led to use this book in order to enhance their care of patients with problematic, puzzling, non-healing wounds. May God bless you all as you work to care for His children!

Rose Hamm and Joseph Carey

Evaluation of the Patient with a Wound

INTRODUCTION

The evaluation of the patient with a non-healing wound consists of the following three components: subjective history, medical history, and wound assessment. The histories usually allows the clinician to make a diagnosis of wound etiology, and if not, at least indicate what needs to be ruled out. Thorough histories also give indications as to why a wound is not healing. The wound assessment provides data for objective, measurable outcomes and progress, as well as information on how to treat the wound initially. The most important aspects of treating any wound are to treat all underlying co-morbidities and to address any issues that may be impeding wound healing. Finally, the initial treatment will consist of appropriate debridement of necrotic tissue and application of a dressing that will ensure adequate moisture for wound healing to advance. Signs and symptoms that suggest the patient be referred to the primary care physician, a medical specialist, or the emergency room are listed in Table 1-1.

TABLE 1-1. Signs and symptoms that suggest a patient be referred to a primary care physician or an emergency room

Sign or Symptom	Suspicious Condition
Erythema, edema, deep pain, hot skin	Necrotizing fasciitis
	Cellulitis
Shortness of breath	Congestive heart failure (CHF)
Lower extremity edema	Renal failure, CHF
Chest pain	Acute MI
Rash, itching, edema, shortness of breath	Drug allergy, drug-induced hypersensitivity syndrome
Blisters and pain along a dermatome	Acute onset of herpes zoster
Dark mole with asymmetry, uneven borders, changing color, more than 1 cm in diameter, and evolving	Melanoma

(Continued)

TABLE 1.1.   Signs and symptoms that suggest a patient be referred to a primary care physician or an emergency room (*Continued*)

Sign or Symptom	Suspicious Condition
Lower extremity pain that increases with activity or awakens the patient at night	Moderate to severe peripheral arterial disease
Syncope, dizziness	Hypotension, hypoglycemia
Decreased mental status	Hypoglycemia, sepsis, cerebral vascular event
Bleeding that is not controlled by pressure	Arterial leak, high INR, low platelet count
New onset of ecchymosis in a distal extremity	Peripheral arterial occlusion
Erythema, warm skin, pain in the foot with weight-bearing in patient with diabetes	Acute Charcot foot
Erythema more than 2 cm beyond the wound border of a diabetic foot ulcer	Infection of the wound
Probe to bone in an exposed wound	Osteomyelitis

SUBJECTIVE HISTORY

Pertinent information to obtain during the subjective interview includes origin and duration of the wound; any notable precipitating events; what treatment has been used (especially what has been used to cleanse and dress the wound); other signs and symptoms such as fever, pruritis, pain levels, and pain description; any co-morbidities such as diabetes, cardiovascular disease, or auto-immune disorders; medications, both prescribed and over-the-counter; allergies; nutritional status; activity level and assistive devices being used; and social habits such as smoking (including vaping), alcohol intake, and drug use. These questions not only assist in making a wound diagnosis, but are imperative for determining *why* the wound is not healing.

MEDICAL HISTORY

The objective medical history is pertinent for co-morbidities, medications, and effective management of skin disorders , as well as any surgeries that may have an impact on the patient's overall well-being. Laboratory values that can be beneficial in determining why a wound is not healing are listed in Table 1-2. Factors, other than co-morbidities, that are known to impede wound healing that need to be monitored and addressed include the following:

- Infection
  - Local
  - Systemic
- Edema
  - Periwound
  - Chronic venous insufficiency

- Medications
  - Steroids
  - Nonsteroidal anti-inflammatory drugs
  - Anticoagulants
  - Antirejection medications
- Nutritional deficits, especially protein malnutrition
- Unrelieved pressure, friction, or shear
- Smoking (including vaping)
- Moderate to heavy alcohol intake
- Stress
- Presence of foreign bodies

TABLE 1-2. Laboratory values with implications for wound healing

Laboratory Test	Normal Range	Values Affecting Wound Healing	Clinical Presentation
CBC			
WBC	$4.5-11 \times 10^3/mm^3$	Increased Decreased	Signs of infection, inflammation, necrosis, trauma, or stress Failure to initiate immune response against bacteria
RBC	M $4.5-5.5 \times 10^6/mm^3$ F $4.1-4.9 \times 10^6/mm^3$	Decreased	Pale or anemic granulation or failure to progress
Hemoglobin	M $13.5-18$ g/dL F $12-15$ g/dL	Decreased Increased	Pale or anemic granulation or failure to progress Failure to progress (patient may show signs of congestive heart failure or COPD)
Hematocrit	M $37-50\%$ F $36-46\%$	Decreased Increased	Pale or anemic granulation or failure to progress in healing Signs of thrombi or emboli
Platelet count	$150-400 \times 10^3/mm^3$	Decreased Increased	Bleeds easily Fatigue Signs Signs of infection or inflammation
Automated Differential			
Neutrophil rel	$57-67\%$ of leukocyte count	Increased	Bacterial infection Chronic inflammation
Lymphocyte rel	$25-33\%$ of leukocyte count	Increased Decreased	Signs of bacterial infection Opportunistic infections

(Continued)

TABLE 1-2.   Laboratory values with implications for wound healing (*Continued*)

Laboratory Test	Normal Range	Values Affecting Wound Healing	Clinical Presentation
Monocyte rel	3−7% of leukocyte count	Increased	Tissue injury Early healing response
Eosinophil rel	1−4% of leukocyte count	Increased Decreased (with corticosteroid use)	Allergic reaction Parasitic infection Delayed inflammatory response
Basophil rel	0−0.75% of leukocyte count	Increased	Allergic reaction
Neutrophil abs	4,300−10,000 cells/mm³	Increased	Signs of infection
Lymphocyte abs	2500−3300 cells/mm³ 2000−2500/μL	Increased Decreased	Signs of bacterial infection Opportunistic infections
Monocyte abs			
Eosinophil abs			
Basophil abs	0−1000 cells/mm³	Increased	Allergic reaction
Coagulation Studies			
PT (prothrombin time)	12.3−14.2 s	Increased (>2.5 × reference range)	Bleeds easily
PTT (partial thromboplastin time)	25−34 s		
INR	Normal 0.9−1.1 Therapeutic range 2−3 Mechanical heart valves 2.5−3.5	Elevated	Bleeds easily Skin bruising
Routine Chemistry			
Sodium	135−145 mEq/L		
Potassium	3.5−5.3 mEq/L		
Chloride	95−105 mEq/L		

TABLE 1-2. Laboratory values with implications for wound healing (*Continued*)

Laboratory Test	Normal Range	Values Affecting Wound Healing	Clinical Presentation
CO_2	22–29 mEq/L 35–45 mmHg (arterial)		
Glucose	70–115 mg/dL	Decreased (<70) Increased (>200)	Headache, dizziness, altered mental status, malaise Arrested healing processed Signs of infection Increased risk of abscess formation
Calcium	8.8–10.5 mg/dL		
Phosphate	2.5–5.0 mg/dL		
BUN	7–18 mg/dL	Increased (renal failure) Decreased (liver failure)	Edema Poor healing Jaundiced skin Yellow fluids
Creatinine	0.1–1.2 mg/dL	Increased (renal failure)	Edema
Albumin	3.5–5.5 g/dL	Decreased Increased	Decreased lean body mass Lack of granulation tissue Bilateral edema Muscle wasting Signs of dehydration
Pre-albumin level	15–36 mg/dL	Decreased	Poor wound healing Lack of granulation formation
Globulin	2.5–3.5 g/dL		
Fibrinogen	200–400 mg/dL		
A/G ratio	1.5:1–2.5:1	Decreased (liver damage) Increased (iron deficiency)	
Bilirubin total	0.1–1.0 mg/dL	Increased	Yellow wound fluids Jaundiced skin
Alkaline phosphate	30–85 U/L		
Others			
HbA1C	4–6%	Increased	Delayed healing

(Continued)

TABLE 1-2. Laboratory values with implications for wound healing (*Continued*)

Laboratory Test	Normal Range	Values Affecting Wound Healing	Clinical Presentation
C-reactive protein	0−1.0 mg/dL or <10 mg/L	Increased	Inflammation Infection
Erythrocyte sedimentation rate (ESR)	Male 0-20 mm/hr Female 0-30 mm/hr (age dependent)	Increased	Infection Inflammation Autoimmune disorder Anemia Poor wound healing
Retinal binding protein	10 mg/L 0.002 g/kg body wt	Increased	Delayed healing due to protein deficits
Magnesium	1.5−2.5 mEq/L		
Phosphorus	2.5-4.5 mg/dL		
Iron		Decreased Increased	Lack of granulation Hemochromatosis
Ferritin		Decreased Increased	Anemic granulation Lack of granulation Hemosiderosis
Transferrin	204−360 µg/dL <0.1 g/kg body wt	Decreased Increased	Delayed wound healing due to protein deficits Iron deficiency
Zinc	>60 µg/dL	Decreased	Delayed wound healing Lack of epithelialization Bullous−pustular dermatitis Intercurrent infections Weight loss
Microbiology			
Wound culture	Negative	Positive	Poor wound healing Wound degradation
Blood culture	Negative	Positive	Systemic signs of infection

Data from Goodman CC, Fuller KS, Boissonnault WG. Pathology: Implications for the Physical Therapist, 2nd ed. Philadelphia, PA: Saunders; 2003 and Huether SE, McCance KL. Understanding Pathophysiology, 4th ed. St Louis, MO: Mosby; 2008.

In lower extremity wounds, lack of adequate circulation is frequently a contributing factor. A complete vascular screening (including pulses, capillary refill, and skin turgor) is advised for any patient with a wound below the knee.[1] *After* the etiology is determined and inhibiting factors are identified, the clinician can address the wound!

WOUND ASSESSMENT

The primary wound assessment that is used by third-party payers to determine efficacy of a treatment plan is the wound size; however, there are other characteristics that may be indicative of wound healing before a reduction in size is observed, including the amount and kind of drainage, pain levels, and type of tissue in the wound bed. Components of the wound assessment include the following:

- Location
- Dimensions
- Undermining and sinuses
- Tissue type
- Drainage (amount and type)
- Periwound skin characteristics
- Periwound sensation (using Semmes-Weinstein monofilaments for patients with diabetes)
- Edema
- Wound edges
- Wound odor
- Signs of infection
- Pain

Characteristics of the four most common types of wounds (arterial, venous, pressure, and diabetic) are described in Table 1-3. Of those, location is one of the most indicative and most frequently over-looked, as will be discussed in the subsequent chapters, along with characteristics that are unique to atypical or unusual wound types. Some of the most common red flags that a wound is not typical are listed in Table 1-4.

INITIAL WOUND TREATMENT

The initial treatment of *almost* all wounds involves (1) debridement of necrotic or infected tissue, (2) treatment of microbes that may be interfering with the wound healing process, and (3) application of a dressing that will maintain adequate moisture balance. Wounds that should *not* be debrided include the following:

- Wounds suspected of being pyoderma grangrenosum (see page 135)
- Wounds with inadequate perfusion for healing
  - 0 or 1+ pulses
  - Ankle brachial index < 0.5
  - Trancutaneous oxygen tension (TcPO$_2$) <30 mmgHg
- Wounds with *non-fluctuant* dry eschar (also termed stable eschar) on the heels of non-ambulatory patients
- Eschar that is adhered to underlying tendons, muscle fibers, or bone

The basic wound care supplies for any office or clinic are listed in Table 1-5. While a complete discussion of sharp debridement techniques is beyond the scope of this chapter, the goal is to remove as much of the non-viable tissue as possible given the

TABLE 1-3. Characteristics of the four typical wound etiologies

Wound Evaluation By Etiology					
	Location	Tissue	Pain	Skin	Exudate
Arterial	Distal digits (toes or fingers)	Dry, necrotic slough, little or no granulation	Yes!!! May have dependent leg syndrome or rest pain	Dry, hairless, shiny, thin, positive rubor of dependency	None unless infected
Venous	Lower 1/3 of the leg (called the gaiter area)	Red or pink, bark-like texture Yellow slough Poor granulation	Generally not painful unless vasculitic or infected	Hemosiderosis (dark, brawny appearance) Atrophie blanche Thick scales	Varies, may have copious serous drainage
Pressure	Over bony prominences	Varies from non-blanchable erythema to dark red to eschar	Varies depending on the structures involved	Discolored from erythematous to hypoxic May be macerated or excoriated	Varies
Neuropathic	Weight-bearing surface of the foot or dorsal digits	Callus or blister, slough, May probe to bone Necrotic if PAD is present	None!!! Until infected, then deep throbbing	Dry, thick, scaly, hyperkeratotic	Varies, depending on infection

Reproduced with permission from Hamm RL: Text and Atlas of Wound Diagnosis and Treatment, 2nd ed. New York, NY: McGraw Hill; 2019.

TABLE 1-4. Characteristics of atypical wounds (not arterial, venous, pressure, or diabetic)

Unusual location
Unusual age of patient
Assymetric lesion
Granulation extending over the wound edges
Exuberant granulation tissue or callus
Friable granulation tissue
Purple-red (violaceous) periwound edges
Ulcer in the center of pigmented lesion
History of repeated trauma
Rolled edges (termed epibole)
Fungating growth
History of radiation therapy
Wound secondary to burns or trauma
No other obvious diagnosis

TABLE 1-5.   Recommended wound care supplies for any clinic or medical office

4x4 gauze pads
Normal saline for cleansing
Debridement kit or suture removal kit with iris scissors and scalpel
Sterile cotton-tipped applicator to measure depth and explore sinuses
Hemostatic agents (e.g. Surgicel)
Measuring guides
Camera for photographs
Dressings as listed in Table 1-7

patient's pain tolerance, with care to protect viable tissues under the eschar and to minimize bleeding.

In cases where pain levels do not allow sharp debridement, autolytic or enzymatic debridement are alternatives; however, the time to convert a chronic wound to an acute wound and thereby facilitate the healing process is much longer with these techniques. At present the only approved enzymatic debridement agent is Collagenase (marketed under the trade name Santyl, Smith & Nephew, Fort Worth, TX) which is best applied daily, but can be applied two to three times a week if dressings do not need to be replaced daily.[2]

If signs of local critical colonization of bacteria are visible, topical antimicrobial dressings [silver, cadexomer iodine, medicinal honey, or polyhexamethylene biguanide (PHMB)] are recommended.[3] Systemic antibiotics should be reserved for patients who have signs and symptoms of infection.[4] Table 1-6 lists signs of infection in a wound for which systemic antibiotics are indicated. In addition, patient conditions that need to be considered when deciding on the use of systemic antibiotics include acquired immunosuppressive disease (e.g. diabetes), severe acquired or innate immunodefeciency (e.g. HIV infection, AIDs, post stem cell transplant), use of immunosuppressant medications, age, or wounds that contain foreign material (e.g. joint replacements).[5]

TABLE 1-6.   Signs of wound infection that suggest the need for systemic antibiotics

Erythema is usually darker than the erythema observed with inflammation; has distinct borders; may streak away from the wound
Pain is usually deep and described as throbbing
Edema is usually with diffuse borders; is localized to the wound site rather than full extremity edema observed with chronic venous insufficiency or lymphedema
Heat is usually palpable as warm periwound skin; may be measured with an infrared skin thermometer with a differential of 3° F considered significant
Purulence is thick exudate due to the bacterial content; may or may not have an odor
Malaise consists of patient complaints of feeling tired and lacking energy; may be accompanied by increased temperature except in patients with diabetes

After appropriate debridement, a dressing is applied that will maintain adequate moisture balance for wound healing to progress (i.e. a moist dressing to a dry wound, an absorbent dressing to a draining wound) without causing maceration to the surrounding skin. Note that wet-to-dry dressings are no longer considered standard care and should only be applied when no other options are available. Table 1-7 lists the

TABLE 1-7.   Basic dressings for initial wound care

Hydrogel (with or without silver)
Cellulose or alginate dressings (with or without silver)
Iodoflex or Iodoform
Xeroform
Silicone-backed foam dressings in a variety of sizes
Transparent film for autolytic debridement
Conforming or cotton gauze rolls for anchoring dressings (2″ and 4″)
Paper tape and hypoallergenic tape
Short-stretch bandages for managing lower extremity edem

TABLE 1-8.   Supplies that are detrimental to wound healing

Betadine
Hydrogen peroxide
Dakin's solution
Acetic acid

basic dressing supplies recommended for any clinic or medical office that sees patients with wounds, and Table 1-8 lists topical agents that are known to be cytotoxic to healthy cells, especially fibroblasts, that are responsible for synthesis of new tissue. Any bandages to manage edema are applied from the distal extremity to the next joint (e.g. below the knee for lower extremity wounds) in a spiral or figure 8 technique in order to avoid creating a tourniquet effect which can increase edema and impede wound healing, as well as cause patient discomfort. Dressings are best applied so that no tape is placed on the skin, especially for patients with thin fragile skin that can tear easily upon removal of the tape. Silicone-backed foam dressings with adhesive borders are recommended for those patients. Any patient whose wound fails to show progress in 2 weeks is advised to be referred to a wound specialist.

Both typical and atypical wounds, along with their pathophysiology, clinical presentation, and recommended medical and wound treatment, are described in the following chapters.

REFERENCES

1. Snyder RJ, Jensen J, Applewhite AJ, Couch K, et al. A standardized approach to evaluating lower extremity chronic wounds using a checklist. *Wounds.* 2019;31(5):S29-S44.
2. Weir D, Scarborough P. Wound debridement. In: Hamm R, ed. *Text and Atlas of Wound Diagnosis and Treatment.* 2nd ed. New York: McGraw Hill Education; 2019;349-371.
3. Weir D, Brindle T. Wound dressings. In: Hamm R, ed. *Text and Atlas of Wound Diagnosis and Treatment.* 2nd ed. New York: McGraw Hill Education; 2019;373-417.
4. Care Partners. Signs, Symptoms and Actions for Superficial and Spreading Wound Infection (All Etiology's). October 2014. Available at wwwoundcare.ca/Uploads/ContentDocuments/ Signs%2C%20Symptoms%20and%20Actions%20for%20Superficial%20and%20 Spreading%20Wound%20Infection%20%28All%20Etiology%27s%29%2C%20Care%20 Partners%2C%20Oct%2020%2C%202014.pdf. Accessed on May 27, 2019.
5. Reitan RL, McBroom RM, Gilder RE. The risk of infection and indication of systemic antibiotics in chronic wounds. *Wounds: A Compendium of Clinical Research and Practice.* 2020;32(7):186-194.

2

Ischemic Wounds

INTRODUCTION

Most ischemic wounds are caused by moderate to severe peripheral arterial disease (PAD); however, there are several systemic disorders that can also cause skin hypo-perfusion which results in non-healing wounds, e.g. arterial entrapment, thrombus, adventitial cyst, embolism, fibromuscular dysplasia, dissection, trauma, vasculitis, and vasospasm.[1] Successful treatment of any ischemic wound depends first upon treatment of the underlying disease, be it PAD or some other malady such as pressure, chronic venous insufficiency, autoimmune diseases, trauma, diabetes, or infection. Evaluation of any wound that presents below the knee *must* include a thorough vascular screening to rule out PAD as a contributing factor. This chapter illustrates ischemic wounds caused by both PAD and systemic disorders, as well as signs and symptoms for a differential diagnosis.

CLASSIFICATION

The American College of Cardiology/American Heart Association Practice Guidelines classify the presentation of PAD into four categories: asymptomatic, claudication, critical limb ischemia, and acute limb ischemia.[2] Frequently the first sign that an *asymptomatic* patient may have PAD is a non-healing wound on the distal foot even though no other symptoms are present. *Claudication* is characterized by fatigue, discomfort, heaviness, or pain in the lower extremities with a predictable amount of exercise; it is relieved by rest and best treated with supervised exercise therapy.[3] *Critical limb ischemia (CLI)*, caused by moderate to severe PAD, is characterized by rest pain, nocturnal recumbent pain, or ischemic lesions that are typically present for at least 2 weeks. *Acute limb ischemia* can occur up to 2 weeks from the onset of symptoms and is characterized by the 6 "Ps"—pain, paralysis, paresthesia, pulselessness, poikilothermia (inability to regulate one's core body temperature), and pallor.[1]

The Society for Vascular Surgery has developed a risk stratification system based on Wound, Ischemia, and foot Infection (WIfI) that takes into account the wound size, the degree of perfusion, and the presence of infection. WIfI is the first PAD tool to take into consideration all three aspects of a lower extremity wound and is especially useful for diabetic foot ulcers which frequently have an arterial component. The WIfI lower extremity threatened limb classification is depicted in Figure 2-1. Although it is used primarily by

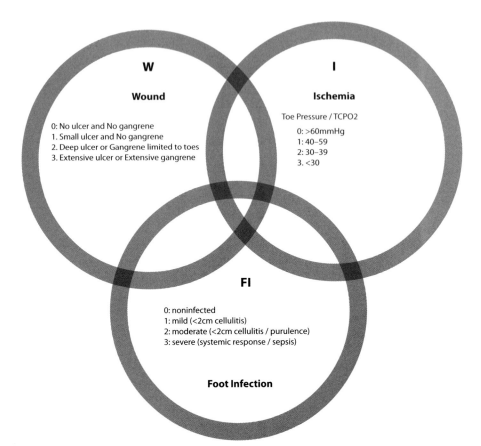

FIGURE 2-1. The Lower Extremity Threatened Limb Classification (WIfI). Wound presence, ischemia, and foot infection are each described and given a numerical value from 0 to 3, and the total number is used to estimate the value of revascularization and the risk for amputation.

Data from Mills JL Sr, Conte MS, Armstrong DG, et al. The Society for Vascular Surgery Lower Extremity Threatened Limb Classification System: risk stratification based on wound, ischemia, and foot infection (WIfI), J Vasc Surg 2014 Jan;59(1):220-234.

vascular surgeons and podiatrists, the WIfI classification can be a useful guide for any clinician in assessing the severity of a patient's condition when presenting with a lower extremity wound. For example, a patient with a small lesion on the foot with palpable pulses and no signs of infection will probably respond to standard wound care as described in Chapter 1. Any patient who has diminished pulses should be referred to a vascular specialist; any patient with signs of infection should be assessed and treated appropriately, with either topical antimicrobial dressings or systemic antibiotics. Table 2-1 lists the signs of local and systemic infection.

ARTERIAL WOUND WITH NO OTHER SYMPTOMS

Figures 2-2 through 2-7

Pathophysiology
- Minor trauma that does not heal in a timely manner due to diminished blood supply as a result of mild to moderate PAD

TABLE 2-1. Signs of local and systemic infection

Local:
- Local swelling or induration
- Erythema between between 0.5 and 2 cm around the wound
- Local tenderness or pain
- Local warmth
- Purulent discharge

Systemic:
- Local infection as described above
- Temperature >38° or <36°
- Heart rate >90 beats/min
- Respiratory rate >20 breaths/min or PaCO$_2$ <32mmHg
- White blood cell count >12,000 or <4000 cu/mm or 10% immature (band) forms

Data from Mills JL Sr, Conte MS, Armstrong DG, et al. The Society for Vascular Surgery Lower Extremity Threatened Limb Classification System: risk stratification based on wound, ischemia, and foot infection (WIfI), J Vasc Surg 2014 Jan;59(1):220-234.

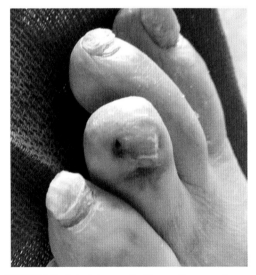

FIGURE 2-2. Arterial wound with no other symptoms.

Clinical presentation
- Minimal tissue loss
- Shallow with no bone or tendon exposed
- Minimal necrotic tissue
- No granulation tissue
- Even edges that create a "punched out" appearance
- Little or no drainage
- Palpable but diminished pulses
- ABI 0.6–0.8, indicative of mild to moderate PAD

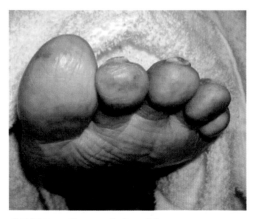

FIGURE 2-3. **Hypoperfusion of the toes.**

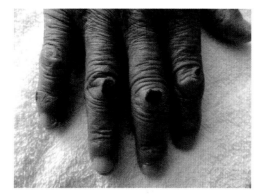

FIGURE 2-4. **Ischemic necrotic wounds on the hand.**

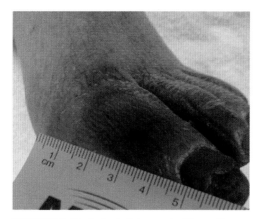

FIGURE 2-5. **Typical arterial wound with no other symptoms; note skin and nail changes.**

- Other signs of arterial disease
  - o Hair loss on the toes
  - o Shiny or scaly skin
  - o Thickened nails
  - o Positive rubor of dependency

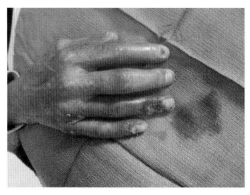

FIGURE 2-6. Ischemic wound on the 4th finger.

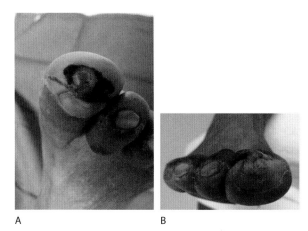

A   B

FIGURE 2-7. (A) Before debridement. (B) After conservative debridement.

Medical management
- Manage co-morbidities often accompanying PAD
  - Diabetes
  - Dyslipidemia
  - Hypertension
  - Hypercholesterolemia
- Monitor progression of PAD
- Consider use of antiplatelet agents (aspirin or clopidogrel)[1]
- Consider use of vasodilators (pentoxyfylline or cilastazol)[1]
- Educate patient to cease smoking or vaping[4]
- Initiate supervised exercise therapy for synthesis of collateral circulation *after* the wound has healed[1]

Wound management
- Cleanse the wound with a non-cytotoxic wound cleanser or tap water; cover with an occlusive dressing
- Avoid aggressive debridement; trim loosened necrotic tissue at the edges as the wound heals

- Determine and remove any source of trauma
- Place foot in an open-toe, post-operative shoe or sandal that will remove all pressure or friction from the affected digit
- Fit in appropriate adaptive shoes after the wound is healed
- For wounds on the hand, treat with standard care as described in Chapter 1 and educate patient to wear protective gloves.

CRITICAL LIMB ISCHEMIA WITH WOUND

Figures 2-8 through 2-11

Pathophysiology
- Severe PAD as a result of an occlusion in the macrovascular system
- Multilevel disease
  - ○ Inflow (iliac, common femoral, or superficial femoral arteries
  - ○ Outflow (tibial arteries)[5]
- Inadequate blood supply to meet the oxygen demand needed for wound healing
- Autonomic dysregulation
- Altered blood viscosity
- Decreased erythrocyte fluidity

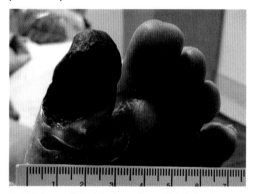

FIGURE 2-8. CLI with signs of possible infection at the base of the great toe (maceration, white blanched skin, peeling epidermis).

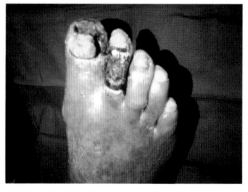

FIGURE 2-9. Well-demarcated necrosis of the 2nd digit (dry gangrene).

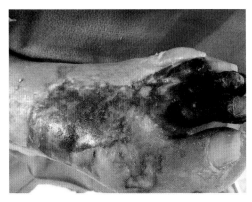

FIGURE 2-10. Necrosis of the toes with signs of diffuse infection (wet gangrene).

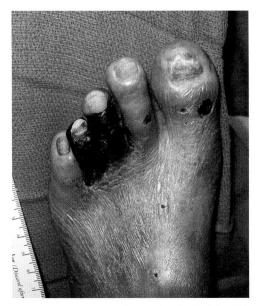

FIGURE 2-11. Necrosis of the 3rd and 4th digits with the typical "punched out" wound on the great toe.

Clinical presentation
- Tissue loss with or without necrosis
- Diminished or absent pulses
- Rest pain, especially at night when in the recumbent position
- Dependent leg syndrome

Medical management
- Immediate referral to a vascular specialist for vascular testing which will guide treatment; healing unlikely without revascularization in the following cases:
  - Toe pressure <55 mmHg[6]
  - Systolic AP <50 mmHg[7]
  - ABI <0.4[7]

- Manage all co-morbidities to optimize wound healing
  - High-dose statin therapy
  - Antiplatelet therapy
  - Antihypertensive therapy[5]
- Treat systemic infection if present
- Limit exercise to functional activities in order to minimize oxygen requirement of lower extremity muscles and thereby increase blood supply to wounded tissue
- Educate patient on importance of smoking cessation
- Monitor perfusion and graft patency (post-revascularization)

Wound management
- Before revascularization
  - Debride only detached or infected tissue
  - Clean edges of eschar with alcohol or betadine solution to decrease bacteria load
  - Place sterile dry gauze or lamb's wool between toes to prevent maceration
  - Use absorbent antimicrobial dressing if there are signs of infection with drainage
- After revascularization
  - *Without surgical debridement*: initiate debridement of necrotic tissue when granulation is visible at the wound edges, a sign of adequate blood flow to the tissue in order for healing to occur
  - *With surgical debridement*: use negative pressure wound therapy (NPWT), moist wound healing, or cellular/tissue product dressings , depending on the size of the wound and the type of tissue present. Delay NPWT until bleeding is controlled.
  - Avoid any elastic compression; if edema is present, use short-stretch, non-elastic wraps
  - Gait train the patient with appropriate off-loading footwear and assistive device
  - Fit with adaptive shoes and inserts (e.g. open-toe post-operative shoe with plastazote inserts) to accommodate any amputation required as well as to prevent pressure at the amputation site during transfers and ambulation

ACUTE LIMB ISCHEMIA

Figures 2-12 through 2-14

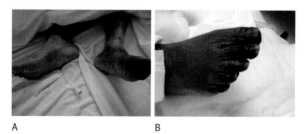

A   B

FIGURE 2-12. (A) Initial signs of acute limb ischemia.
(B) Progression observed one week later.

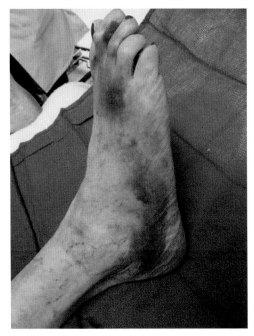

FIGURE 2-13. Embolic acute limb ischemia.

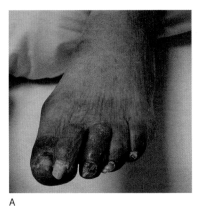 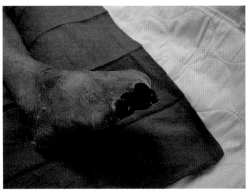

A   B

FIGURE 2-14. A. Acute limb ischemia in which the tissue is not yet demarcated. B. Demarcated tissue necrosis after acute limb ischemia.

Pathophysiology
- Emergent precipitous decrease in limb perfusion that threatens the viability of the limb distal to the occlusion, of less than 14 days duration
  - Thrombotic: history of PAD, evidence of tissue hypoperfusion occurs within hours to days
  - Embolic: history of atrial fibrillation or prosthetic heart valve; acute onset of complete occlusion without opportunity for collateral vessel development; patient may report absolute time of onset; embolism occurs at site of vessel bifurcation[8]

Clinical presentation
- Six Ps: pain, pallor, paresthesia, paralysis, pulselessness, and poikilothermic
- Mottled or marbled skin
- ABI < 0.5

Medical management
- Refer immediately to a vascular specialist
- Place extremity in a dependent position
- Administer IV heparin bolus (100 U/kg followed by continuous infusion of 1000 U/hr until INR is 2 to 3)[8]
- Follow with constant IV infusion of heparin[8]
- Monitor for reperfusion injury, major bleeding at other sites, and compartment syndrome

Wound management
- No wound management indicated, even with tissue necrosis, until medical treatment is completed and tissue viability is well-demarcated. Distal digits that become necrotic and demarcated may auto-amputate.

COMPARTMENT SYNDROME

Figures 2-15 through 2-19

Pathophysiology
- Increased pressure within an anatomical compartment that results in inadequate perfusion of the enclosed tissue. May be associated with any of the following conditions:
  - Drug or alcohol related episodes that result in prolonged immobility[9,10]
  - Prolonged immobility during surgery, e.g. in the lithotomy or hemi-lithotomy position[11]
  - Post-trauma or fracture
- Frequently associated with rhabdomyolysis
- Increased expansive force from edema with resulting increased venous pressure, venous occlusion, and eventual decreased arterial perfusion[10]
- Tissue necrosis as a result of hypo-perfusion

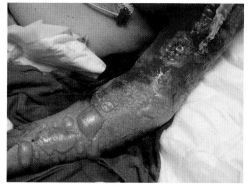

FIGURE 2-15. Compartment syndrome of the upper extremity after shoulder surgery.

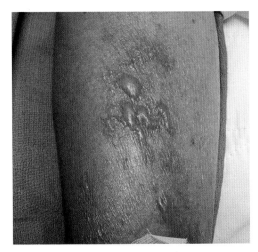

FIGURE 2-16. Initial presentation of compartment syndrome may involve blistering.

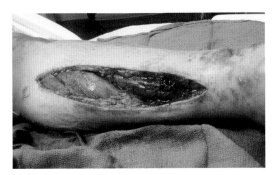

FIGURE 2-17. After fasciotomy; non-viable muscle has to be debrided.

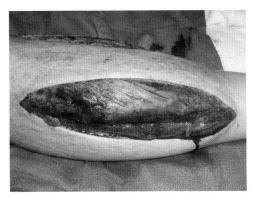

FIGURE 2-18. After fasciotomy, bleeding needs to be controlled before applying NPWT.

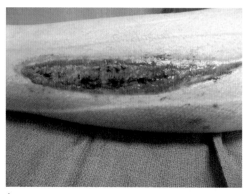

A

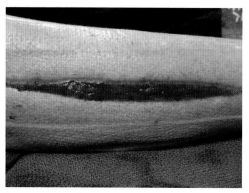

B

FIGURE 2-19. (A) Fasciotomy after NPWT. (B) Wound ready for transition to moist wound healing to promote epithelial migration or for application of split-thickness skin graft.

Clinical presentation
- Usually occurs in anterior compartment of the lower leg, but may also occur in the thigh, buttock, forearm, hand, shoulder, or foot
- Presents with 6 Ps: pain, paresthesia, pallor, paralysis, diminished pulses or capillary refill, and increased intra-compartmental pressure (>30 mmHg in normotensive patients; >20 mmHg in hypotensive patients)[10]
- Presents with hard edema, tenderness with palpation, and erythema around the affected tissue
- Increased serum creatinine kinase[10]

> **Diagnostic Clue:** Acute compartment syndrome is differentiated from chronic or exertional compartment syndrome which occurs in the lower leg with a predictable amount of strenuous exercise especially in "weekend" athletes who do not train and stretch properly.

Medical management
- Emergent fasciotomy, preferably within the first 6 hours
- Resuscitation
- Management of co-morbidities

Wound management
- Negative pressure wound therapy post fasciotomy
- Skin graft or cellular/tissue therapy when fully granulated

---

Diagnostic Clue: If a wound appears arterial in origin but on the lower extremity of a younger person who would not be expected to have arterial disease, it is probably atypical in origin and other pathological processes need to be explored.

THROMBOANGIITIS OBLITERANS/BUERGER'S DISEASE

Figures 2-20 and 2-21

Pathophysiology
- Is a non-atherosclerotic inflammatory disease of the small- and medium-sized vessels of the extremities
- Is strongly associated with smoking, primarily in men under 50 years of age
- Is characterized by hypercellular inflammatory thrombus with minimal inflammation in the vessel wall, progressing to thrombus with vascular fibrosis and vasospasm
- Has predominantly polymorphonuclear (PMN) leukocytes at the site of inflammation[12]

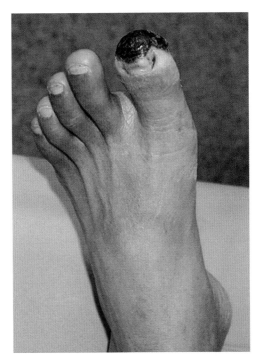

FIGURE 2-20. Thromboangiitis obliterans on the foot of a young male.

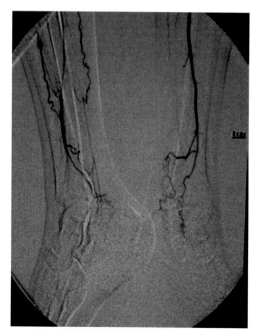

FIGURE 2-21. Arterial radiograph illustrates vasospasm that results in tissue ischemia on the distal great toe.

Clinical presentation
- Thin, shiny skin distal to the occlusion
- Thickened malformed nails
- Dusky, cool, and painful digits[13]
- Tissue necrosis of distal digits (in advanced stage)
- Positive Allen's test (for the hand)[13]
- Possible Raynaud's phenomenon

Medical management
- Smoking cessation
- Avoid nicotine substitutes[13]
- Vascular referral for possible revascularization or endovascular procedure
- Vasodilators if occlusion is not complete[13]

Wound management
- Protection of digits from pressure or maceration
- Debride only when deemed advisable based on vascular studies

CARDIAC DISEASE

Figures 2-22 and 2-23

Pathophysiology
- Decreased flow of blood to the wounded area, especially distally
- Decreased oxygen and nutrients carried to the wounded tissue
- Decreased cardiac output and concurrent peripheral edema associated with congestive heart failure (CHF)

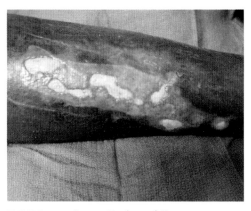

FIGURE 2-22. Congestive heart failure.

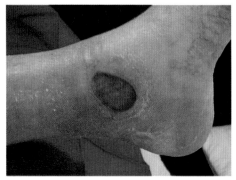

A

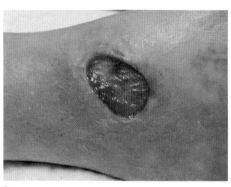

B

FIGURE 2-23. (A) Occluded coronary arteries, before CABG. (B) Note little change in granulation after 3 weeks of standard care, before CABG.

Clinical presentation
- Usually occurs on distal extremities
- May have another etiology (e.g. pressure, trauma, venous insufficiency) but does not respond to standard care
- Has the appearance of an ischemic wound, i.e. round even edges, poor granulation tissue, minimal drainage[14]
- May be painful

Medical management
- Manage cardiac risk factors (hypertension, hypercholesterolemia)
- Manage co-morbidities that contribute to cardiac disease (e.g. diabetes)
- Educate about smoking cessation
- Administer appropriate diuretics for CHF
- Assess for cardiac revascularization

Wound management
- Standard moist wound care
- Conservative debridement if needed (autolytic or enzymatic)
- Compression for LE edema due to CHF (confirm with cardiologist when compression is safe and the amount of compression that can be tolerated without overloading the heart)

PURPURA FULMINANS

Figures 2-24 through 2-27

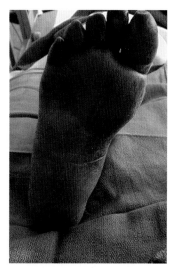

FIGURE 2-24. Purpura fulminans of the forefoot.

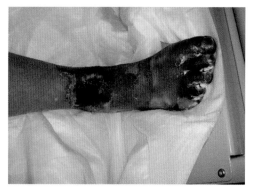

FIGURE 2-25. Purpura fulminans of the entire foot and ankle.

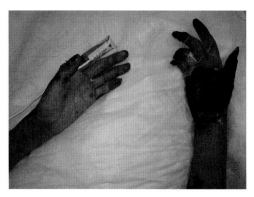

FIGURE 2-26. Purpura fulminans of the hands.

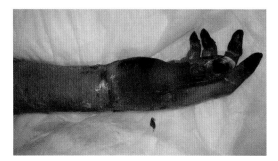

FIGURE 2-27. Side view of the right hand.

Pathophysiology
- Is caused by thrombotic occlusion of the small and medium vessels that leads to skin necrosis
- Occurs with severe sepsis or as an autoimmune response to otherwise benign childhood infections[15]
- May be the presenting symptom of severe inheritable deficiency of the natural anticoagulants protein C or protein S[15]
- May be caused by dysfunction of the protein-C thrombomodulin pathway that exerts a negative effect on coagulation[16]
- May lead to disseminated intravascular coagulation (DIC) with a high mortality rate[16]
- Reported bacterial infections leading to acute infectious PF include *Neisseria meningitides, Streptococcus pneumoniae, Haemophilus influenza, Streptococcus species, Staphylococcus aureus, Capnocytophaga canimorsus,* and *Enterobacter aerogenes*[17]

Clinical presentation
- Presents as hemorrhagic and ecchymotic lesions with skin necrosis
- Usually occurs on the extremities, but may occur on any location
- Is accompanied by high grade fever, chills, and nausea
- Has systemic signs of hypotension and tachycardia
- Also presents with cold limbs, cyanosis, tachypnea[17]

Medical management
- Neonatal management
  - ○ Acute phase: replacement therapy with fresh frozen plasma or protein C concentrate
  - ○ Maintenance therapy: anticoagulation with warfarin or low molecular weight heparin[18]
- Adult management
  - ○ IV fluid resuscitation
  - ○ Antibiotics for the underlying infection
  - ○ Vasopressors
  - ○ Aggressive anticoagulation therapy[16]
  - ○ Platelet transfusions aimed at correcting acquired deficiencies in natural anticoagulant proteins[16]
  - ○ Hemodialysis
  - ○ May require selective amputation

Wound management
- Moist wound healing
- Initial application of hyperoxygenated fatty acids every 2 hours followed by moist wound healing[19] (reported on pediatric patients)
- Palliative wound care in terminal cases

MARTORELL'S ULCER

Figures 2-28 through 2-30

Pathophysiology
- Systemic arterial hypertension that causes obstruction of the small arterioles of the medial artery[20]
- Skin necrosis as a result of ischemia
- Sometimes triggered by trauma, or may be spontaneous
- Prevalence greater in women than in men, age 50–70 years

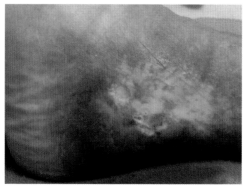

FIGURE 2-28. Martorell's ulcer occurs lower than the typical venous wound.

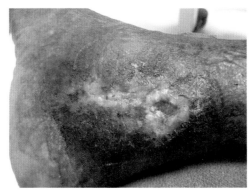

FIGURE 2-29. Martorell's ulcer with satellite lesions.

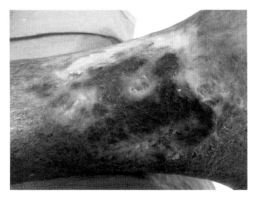

FIGURE 2-30. Thick scarring with Martorell's lesions.

Clinical presentation
- Location on the medial side of the distal third of the lower leg
- Variable depth, necrotic base, and violaceous edges
- Possible presence of satellite lesions
- Diastolic arterial hypertension in the lower limb
- Complaints of severe pain that is increased in the horizontal position
- Absence of arterial calcification or chronic venous insufficiency
- Symmetrical lesions or scarring on the inner side of the distal limb without a wound
- Poor response to treatment[20]

Medical management
- Antihypertensive therapy, especially drugs that reduce vasoconstriction (e.g. calcium channel blockers and ACE inhibitors)[20]
- Smoking cessation
- Education to avoid trauma

Wound management
- Debridement (possibly surgical due to pain levels)
- Moist wound dressings
- Management of edema, if present, with short stretch bandages initially or 25–30 mmHg compression stockings (based on patient tolerance)[20]

REFERENCES

1. Gardner AW, Afaq A. Management of lower extremity peripheral arterial disease. *J Cardiopulm Rehabil Prev.* 2008;28(6):349-357.
2. Hardman RL, Jazaeri O, Yi J, Smith M, Gupta R. Overview of classification systems in peripheral arterial disease. *Seminars in Interventional Radiology.* 2014;31(4):378-388.
3. Jewell DV, Shishehbor MH, Walsworth MK. Centers for Medicare and Medicaid Services policy regarding supervised exercise for patients with intermittent claudication: The good, the bad, and the ugly. *Journal of Orthopaedic & Sports Physical Therapy.* 2017;47(12):892-894
4. Alanazi H, Park HJ, Chakir J, Semlali A, Rouabhia M. Comparative study of the effects of cigarette smoke and electronic cigarettes on human gingival fibroblast proliferation, migration, and apoptosis. *Food Chem Toxicol.* 2018;118:390–398.
5. Shishehbor MH, White CJ, Gray BH, Menard MT, Lookstein R, Resenfield K, Jaff MR. Critical limb ischemia: An expert statement. *Journal of the American College of Cardiology.* 2016;68(18). doi:10.1016/j.jacc.2016.04.071. Accessed August 6, 2019.
6. Mills J, Andros G. Noninvasive assessment of lower extremity hemodynamics in individuals with diabetes. *Journal of Vascular Surgery.* 2010;52(suppl):76S-80S.
7. Mills JL, Conte MS, Armstrong DG, Pomposelli FB, Schanzer A, Sidawy AN, Andros G. The Society for Vascular Surgery lower extremity threatened limb classification system: Risk stratification based on Wound, Ischemia, and foot Infection (WIfI). *Journal of Vascular Surgery.* 2014;59(1):220-234.
8. Baker S, Diercks DB. Acute limb arterial ischemia. *Emergency Medicine.* 2018;50(3):65-71.
9. Rao SS, Mawn G, Lobaton GO, Puvanesrajah V, Amin RM, Humbyrd CJ, Sterling RS. Opioid-related compartment syndrome and associated morbidity. *Injury.* 2019;50(8):1429-1432.
10. Elkbuli A, Sanchez C, Hai S, McKenny M, Boneva D. Gluteal compartment syndrome following alcohol intoxication: Case report and literature review. *Annals of Medicine and Surgery.* 2019;44:98-101.
11. Clarke D, Mullings S, Franklin S, Jones K. Well leg compartment syndrome. *Trauma Case Reports.* 2017;11:5-7.
12. Rivera-Chavarria IJ, Brenes-Gutierrez JD. Thromboangiitis obliterans (Buerger's disease). *Annals of Medicine and Surgery.* 2016;7:79-82.
13. Seebald J, Gritters L. Thromboangiitis obliterans (Buerger disease). *Radiology Case Reports.* 2015;10(3):9-11.
14. Hamm RL, Luttrell T. Factors that impede wound healing. In: Hamm R, ed. *Text and Atlas of Wound Diagnosis and Treatment.* 2nd ed. New York: McGraw-Hill Education; 2019;321-346.
15. Chalmers E, Cooper P, Forman K, Grimley C, Khair K, Minford A, Morgan M, Mumford AD. Purpura fulminans: recognition, diagnosis and management. *Arch Dis Child.* 2011;96(11):1066-1071.
16. Colling ME, Bendapudi PK. Purpura fulminans: Mechanism and management of dys-regulated hemostasis. *Transfusion Medicine Reviews.* 2018;32(2):69-76.
17. Yamamota S, Ito R. Acute infectious purpura fulminans with *Enterobacter aerogenes* post neurosurgery. *Infectious Disease Cases.* 2019;15:e00514. doi:10.1016/j.idcr.2019.e00514. Accessed August 18, 2019.
18. Price VE, Ledingham DL, Krumpel A, Chan AK. Diagnosis and management of neonatal purpura fulminans. *Seminars in Fetal and Neonatal Medicine.* 2011;16(6):318-322.
19. Perez-Acevedo G, Torra-Bou JE, Manzano-Canillas ML, Bosch-Alcaraz A. Management of purpura fulminans skin lesions in a premature neonate with sepsis: a case study. *Journal of Wound Care.* 2019;28(4):198-203.
20. Pinto APFL, Silva NA, Osorio CT, Rivera LM, Carneiro S, Ramos-e-Silva M, Bica BERG. Martorell's ulcer: Diagnostic and therapeutic challenge. *Case Rep Dermatol.* 2015;7(2):199-206.

3

Venous Wounds

INTRODUCTION

Edema in the interstitial tissue around any wound, regardless of etiology, inhibits the healing process by trapping necrotic cells and debris and thereby preventing access of red blood cells to the injured tissue, which in turn decreases the supply of oxygen and nutrients needed for the wound to heal. Management of the edema around a wound depends on the etiology, the location, and the arterial perfusion of the periwound tissue. Determining the etiology of the edema requires a medical and pharmacologic history, surgical history (including type and access points), and joint range of motion and muscle strength in the involved extremities. In addition, evaluation of any lower extremity with edema includes a comprehensive vascular assessment. This chapter discusses wounds caused by or associated with edema, primarily in the lower extremities.

CHRONIC VENOUS INSUFFICIENCY

Figures 3-1 through 3-12

Many lower extremity wounds with edema are caused by chronic venous insufficiency (CVI); however, multiple other etiologies are possible. (See Table 3-1.) Medications that may cause edema are presented in Table 3-2. The focus of treating edema is to eliminate the cause when possible and to apply compression; however, not all compression is the same and trained personnel are recommended for compression application in order to obtain the best outcomes. Figure 3-1 presents an algorithm that is helpful in determining the cause of the edema and *what* to wrap, and Figure 3-2 presents an algorithm for determining the *amount* of compression that can be safely applied to the lower extremity based upon the vascular status. These guidelines are especially imperative for wounds that are a result of combined arterial and venous insufficiency (CAVI). (Figure 3-3) The same principles can apply to upper extremity edema[1] which is also treated with compression wraps; however, short stretch bandages are usually recommended. (Figure 3-4) When the edema extends to the toes and fingers, the digits are incorporated into the compression bandaging using bi-layered gauze rolls.

TABLE 3-1.   Causes of lower extremity edema

Chronic venous insufficiency
Congestive heart failure
Ankle hypomobility
     Fracture
     Sprain/strain
     Rheumatoid arthritis
Immobility
     Spinal cord injuries
     Hemiplegia
Trauma
Infection
Lymphedema
Post-surgical complication
     Hip/knee replacement
     Revascularization procedure
Systemic disorders
     Liver failure
     Renal failure
Obstructed lymph nodes due to malignancy
Medications

CHRONIC VENOUS INSUFFICIENCY (CVI)

Figures 3-5 through 3-12

Pathophysiology
Pathophysiology of CVI can be multi-factorial, involving any of the following pathological disorders:
- Incompetent valves in the superficial or deep veins, resulting in venous reflux
- Deep vein thrombosis resulting in venous occlusion (Figures 3-5)
- Ankle hypomobility resulting in ineffective venous pump (i.e. no gastrocsoleus contraction to compress deep veins and thereby facilitate the pressure gradient between the deep and superficial vessels)
- Inflammation within the venous system with increased hydrostatic pressure that results in increased ambulatory pressure[2]
- Risk factors
  - Varicose veins
  - History of DVT
  - History of vein surgery
  - Family history
  - Female gender
  - Multiple pregnancies
  - Hormone replacement therapy
  - Prolonged standing
  - Sitting postures
  - Obesity[3]
  - Age over 50
  - Factor 5 Leiden mutation[4]

TABLE 3-2.   Medications that may contribute to peripheral edema

Anti-arrhythmics (amniodorone, Norpace, Flecainide)
Anti-coagulants (Plavix, Crestor, Lipitor, Arixtra, Cilostazol)
Antidepressants
Antifungals (Amphoteriicin)
Antihypertensive (nitrates, hydralazine, minoxidil)
Anti-neoplastic (Xeloda, Aromasin, Herceptin, Zometa)
Anti-osteroporotic agents (Actonel, Bisphosphates)
Antisympathetics (reserpine, guanethidine)
Beta- blockers (Tenormin, Coreg, Labetalol, Toprol)
Calcium Channel blockers (Verapamil, Nifedipine)
Chemotherapy agents (docetaxel, cisplatin, trentinion)
Centrally acting agents (clonidine, methyldopa)
Corticosteroids
Direct vasodilators (hydralazine, minoxidil, diazoxide)
Glitazones, Actos, Avandia (DM)
Hormones (Estrogens/progesterones/testosterone)
Nonsteroidal anti-inflammatory agents
Nonselective cyclooxygenase inhibitors
Selective cyclooxygenase-2 inhibitors
Troglitazone
Phenylbutazone
Parkinson agents (Mirapex)
Valproic acid

Data from Cho S, Atwood JE. Peripheral edema, Am J Med 2002 Nov;113(7):580-586.

Clinical presentation
- Patient complaints
  - Heavy feeling in the legs
  - Aching or limb fatigue
  - Symptom relief with elevation
- Skin changes
  - Visible spider veins that may progress to varicose veins
  - Hemosiderosis (Figure 3-6)
  - Atrophie blanche (Figure 3-7)
  - Lipodermatosclerosis (Figure 3-8)
  - Brawny edema
  - Hyperpigmentation

- Chronic wounds
  - Location in the lower third of the extremity (Figure 3-9)
  - Serpentine or irregular edges
  - Gradual onset with enlargement if not treated
  - Shallow fibrotic or poorly-granulated wound base
  - Serous to seropurulent drainage, depending on amount of edema and presence of infection
  - Little to no wound pain (unless there is an arterial component or infection)

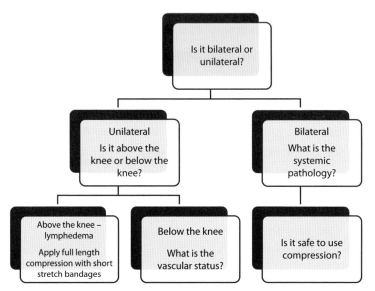

FIGURE 3-1. Algorithm for determining the cause of edema and deciding what to compress.

Compression selection begins with a definitive diagnosis of the edema pathology. If the patient has bilateral lower extremity edema, systemic disorders such as congestive heart failure, kidney failure, or liver disease must be ruled out, in addition to carefully reviewing the medications. If the patient has acute congestive heart failure, compression may need to be deferred until the patient is diuresed and there is no risk of over-loading the heart. Any systemic issue must be addressed in order for local treatment to be effective.

If the edema extends above the knee, there is probably secondary lymphedema which would be treated with manual lymphatic drainage, exercise, and compression applied from toe to upper thigh, preferably by a certified lymphedema specialist. If the edema is limited to below the knee, the next step is to evaluate the vascular status to determine the type of material and the amount of compression that is best for the individual patient. (Used with permission from Rose Hamm)

Diagnostic Clue: Atophie blanche (AB) is a common clinical sign in patients with CVI, and may occur around existing or healing wounds on the distal third of the lower extremity. However, AB may also be the result livedoid vasculopathy, a thrombo-occlusive disorder associated with other conditions (e.g. hyperhomocysteinemia, factor V Leiden mutation, protein C deficiency, lupus-type anticoagulant, and cryoglobulinemia). AB due to livedoid vasculopathy typically occurs in the ankle region and may extend to the dorsum of the foot.[5] (Figure 3-10 and 3-11)

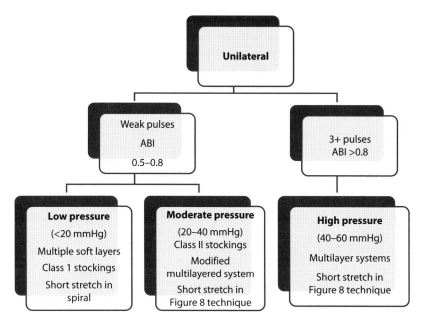

FIGURE 3-2. **Algorithm for selection of appropriate compression therapy.**

Selection of the appropriate compression therapy is based on the vascular examination, as well as patient comfort and tolerance. Every garment, compression system, elastic or non-elastic wrap has a tension that determines the amount of pressure when properly applied. Manufacturer's guidelines should be followed carefully to avoid complications that can occur with inappropriate compression therapy. Compression of any type is generally contraindicated if the ABI is less than 0.5; however, if the patient can tolerate multiple layers of soft gauze wrapping, it may be beneficial in activating the lymphatics as well as anchoring the appropriate primary dressing. Any compression is best applied by a trained professional until the wound is closed and the patient is ready to transition to compression stockings.

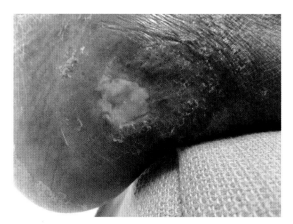

FIGURE 3-3. **Wound due to CAVI.**

Medical management

- Arterial assessment, pulse exam, and ABI[3]
- Venous duplex studies to confirm DVT
- Anticoagulation therapy for acute DVT

- Wound culture only if clinical evidence of infection is present[3]
  - Quantitative bacteriology swabs to identify superficial bacteria
  - Deep wound tissue cultures for wounds with multiple microbes, biofilm, or persistent infection that does not respond to antimicrobial therapy
  - Wound biopsy for wounds that do not respond to standard care after 4–6 weeks of standard care
- Treatment of infection if present
- Pentoxifylline (400 mg 3 times daily for up to 6 months)[6]
- Avoid or discontinue non-steroidal anti-inflammatory medications
- Avoid diuretics unless necessary for other pathologies[9]
- Physical therapy referral for ankle mobilization, gastrocnemius strengthening exercises and gait training to optimize the venous pump

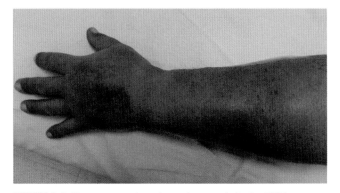

FIGURE 3-4. **Upper extremity edema due to subclavian DVT.**

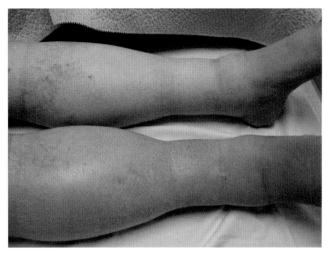

FIGURE 3-5. **Right lower extremity edema due to DVT.**

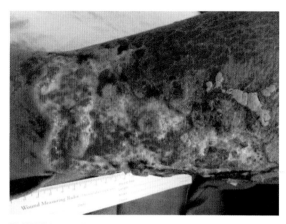

FIGURE 3-6. Full thickness wounds and hemosiderosis due to CVI.

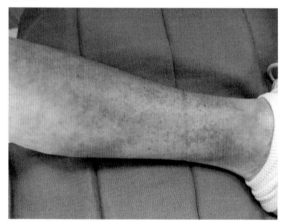

FIGURE 3-7. Atrophie blanche due to CVI.

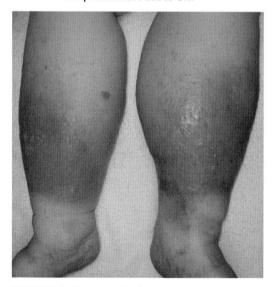

FIGURE 3-8. Lipodermatosclerosis.

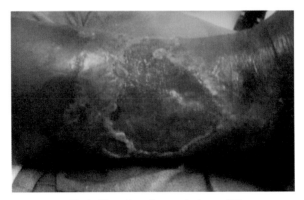

FIGURE 3-9. Typical location of wounds due to CVI.

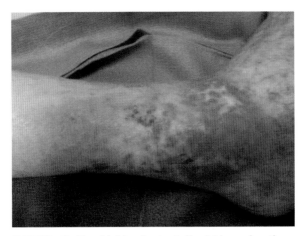

FIGURE 3-10. Atrophie blanche due to livedoid vasculopathy.

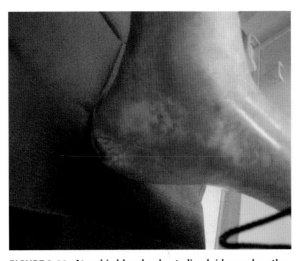

FIGURE 3-11. Atrophie blanche due to livedoid vasculopathy.

Wound management
- Debride necrotic tissue (Figures 3-12 and 3-13)
- Absorbent dressings to manage drainage
- Application of skin lubricants underneath compression bandages
- Application of topical steroids to reduce symptoms of dermatitis that may develop under bandages
- Application of antifungal cream if fungus develops under bandages
- Compression wrap (multi-layer recommended over single-component bandages)[3,7]
- Transition to compression stockings when wounds are closed and remodeling
- Adjunctive therapies if not improved after 4–6 weeks
  - Ultraviolet C for bactericidal effects,
  - Non-contact low-frequency ultrasound to facilitate healing[8,9]
  - Cellular/tissue therapy to facilitate wound closure on clean and granulating wounds
  - Intermittent pneumatic compression when other compression options are not tolerated or available

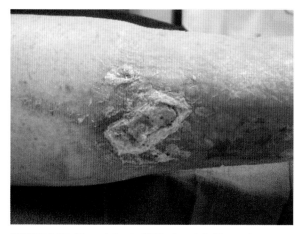

FIGURE 3-12. Wound due to CVI before debridement.

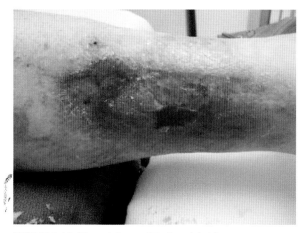

FIGURE 3-13. Wound due to CVI after debridement.

CONGESTIVE HEART FAILURE
Figures 3-14 and 3-15

Pathophysiology
- Ventricular failure
- Arrythmia
- Coronary artery disease
- Valvular disease

Clinical presentation
- Bilateral lower extremity pitting edema
- Associated jugular venous distention and crackles
- Positive brain natriuretic peptide measurement[10]

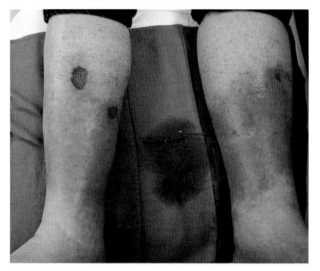

FIGURE 3-14. Lower extremities of a patient with congestive heart failure.

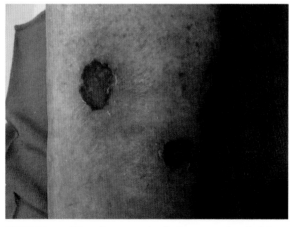

FIGURE 3-15. Wounds as a result of edema associated with congestive heart failure.

Medical management
- Refer to cardiac specialist
- Determine source of heart failure
- Treat other co-morbidities (e.g. diabetes)
- Consider multiple medications recommended by specialist, and their implications
  - Diuretics
  - Anti-hypertensive medications
  - Afterload reducers
  - Anti-coagulation therapies
  - Anti-arrhytmia medications

Wound management
- Moist wound therapy with antimicrobial primary dressings if wound appears critically colonized
- Compression therapy as tolerated once patient is diuresed

LYMPHEDEMA (PRIMARY AND SECONDARY)

Figures 3-16 through 3-18

Pathophysiology
- Primary lymphedema
  - Congenital malformation of the lymphatic system
- Secondary lymphedema
  - Impaired venous flow that results in overload to the lymphatic system
  - Acquired damage to the lymphatic vessels
  - Impaired reabsorption and/or transportation of lymphatic fluid[11]
  - Systemic disorders (e.g. liver, kidney, or cardiac disease)

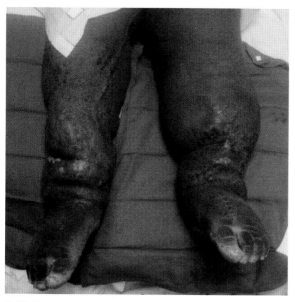

FIGURE 3-16. **Primary lymphedema.**

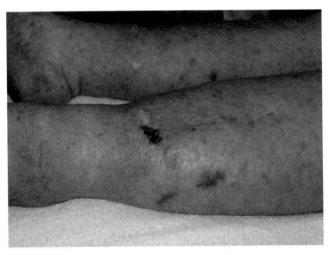

FIGURE 3-17. Secondary lymphedema due to CVI.

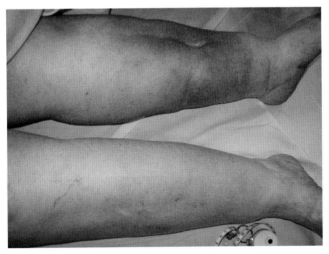

FIGURE 3-18. Secondary lymphedema due to trauma.

- o Medication (see Table 3-2)[10,12]
- o Oncology treatment (e.g. radiation, lymph node dissection)
- o Trauma that disrupts the venous or lymphatic systems
- o Hip or knee surgery that disrupts lymphatic flow and may temporarily decrease venous pump action

Clinical presentation
- • Primary or secondary lymphedema
  - o Stage 0: complaints of heaviness, tightness, or sensory changes in the limb; edema is not evident
  - o Stage 1: variable edema that decreases with rest, sleep, or elevation; increases with activity; soft pitting edema with little or no fibrosis
  - o Stage 2: edema does not dissipate with elevation; positive for fibrosis; may be pitting or non-pitting; brawny skin color; positive Stemmer sign

○ Stage 3: increased fibrosis with little or no skin mobility; coarse or absent hair follicles; hard palpation with little or no pitting; positive Stemmer sign; recurrent infections; unrecognizable limb shape

Medical management

- Optimization of venous and lymphatic flow through exercise and compression therapy in order to prevent secondary lymphedema (if not already present)
- Exercise therapy (see Table 3-3)
- Manual lymphatic mobilization (by a lymphedema specialist)
- Multilayer compression therapy with short-stretch bandages (by a lymphedema specialist)
- Intermittent compression pumps
- Compression garments after lymphedema is maximally reduced
- Skin care (proper cleansing and moisturizing)
- Patient education to avoid restrictive clothing and weight gain
- Consider referral to plastic surgeon with microvascular expertise for lymph node transfer, lymphatic bypass, resection of tissue, liposuction[13,14,15]

TABLE 3-3. Exercise programs for the upper extremity and lower extremity

Upper extremity
Diaphragmatic breathing
Abdominal exercises
Neck rotations
Shoulder circles

Shoulder -> hand
    Pectoralis major ex (PNF diagonal D1, horizontal humeral adduction)
    Scapular adduction (rowing, scapular retraction)
    Latissimus (modified pull-down)
    Internal/external rotation
    Forward flexion to 90°
    Elbow flexion/ext
    Wrist flex/ext/circles
    Finger flex/ext/abd/add
Begin the exercises for the upper extremity by working from the shoulder to the hand, then work distal to proximal with emphasis on shoulder rotation, circles, and breathing.

Lower extremity
Diaphragmatic breathing
Abdominal exercises
Neck rotations
Shoulder circles
Gluteal exercises (bridging)
Inguinal lymph node stimulation (knee to chest)
Ant/post/lat/med thigh ex (open chain SLR in all 4 planes)
Knee flex/ext
Ankle (ankle pumps, circumduction)

(Continued)

TABLE 3-3.   Exercise programs for the upper extremity and lower extremity (*Continued*)

Progress to closed chain exercises
  Marching in place
  Modified squats
  Heel/toe raises
  Modified lunges
  Side-stepping
  Grapevine side to side
  Walking backward
End with inguinal node stimulation and diaphragmatic breathing.

Wound management
- Debridement of necrotic tissue
- Absorbent dressings to manage drainage
- Application of skin lubricants underneath compression bandages
- Application of topical steroids to reduce symptoms of dermatitis that may develop under bandages
- Application of antifungal cream if fungus develops under bandages

LIPEDEMA

Figures 3-19 and 3-20

Pathophysiology
- Abnormal deposition of subcutaneous fat and edema in the lower or upper extremities
- A genetic estrogen-related disorder that affects primarily females
- Not associated with obesity, although there may be clinical overlap with a high BMI and disproportionate weight below the waist[16]
- Onset usually after puberty or after other times of hormonal changes (pregnancy, menopause)[12]

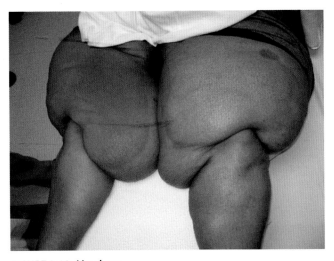

FIGURE 3-19. Lipedema.

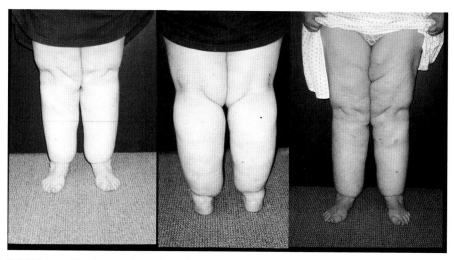

FIGURE 3-20. Lipedema at time of initial diagnosis and after treatment.

From Perdomo M, Hamm RL. Lymphedema. In Hamm RL, ed. Text and Atlas of Wound Diagnosis and Treatment. New York: McGraw-Hill Education. 2019;145-169. Used with permission.

Clinical presentation
- Edema and subcutaneous fat deposits in the lower extremities that usually end just above the ankles
- Bilateral and symmetrical distribution
- Skin folds at the distal edge of the edema (termed positive "cuff sign")[12]
- Complaints of pain, tenderness, and easy bruising[17]
- Irregular skin surface with subcutaneous fatty nodules

Medical management
- Combined decongestive therapy and manual lymphatic drainage
- Compression therapy
- Functional mobilization/exercise[12]
- Liposuction performed under tumescent local anesthesia[18]
- Treat concomitant obesity if present

Wound management
- Standard wound care as described for venous wounds

ACUTE OBSTRUCTION OF LYMPH NODES
Figures 3-21

Diagnostic Clue: Sudden onset of hard, non-pitting edema with no response to compression is an indication that the patient has inguinal lymph node obstruction, and is of immediate concern for an undiagnosed malignancy. Referral to a vascular specialist and/or oncologist is advised.

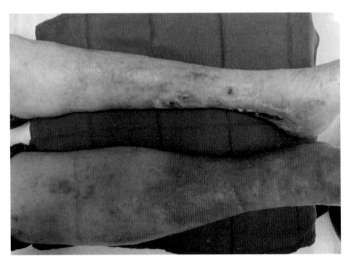

FIGURE 3-21. Right LE Lymphedema due to inguinal lymph node obstruction.
Reproduced with permission from Hamm RL: Text and Atlas of Wound Diagnosis and Treatment, 2nd ed. New York, NY: McGraw Hill; 2019.

Pathophysiology
- Occlusion of lymph nodes as a result of an internal malignancy, resulting in severe lymphedema that does not respond to standard lymphedema care

Clinical presentation
- Hard, painful edema in the extremity distal to the involved lymph nodes
- Often sudden onset as compared to the gradual worsening that occurs with secondary lymphedema
- Variable changes in skin color

Medical management
- Treat the underlying malignancy[19]

Wound management
- Manage any drainage from the skin or open areas with absorbent dressings
- Avoid compression until underlying disease is managed

POST-SURGICAL EDEMA

Figures 3-22 and 3-23

Pathophysiology
- Interruption of the lymphatic flow either at the nodes or the vessels due to the surgical procedure, especially with surgical incisions in the groin and popliteal region[20,21]
- Intraoperative blood loss with or without coagulated hematoma
- Extra-pelvic hematoma causing extravascular compression of the external iliac vein[22]
- Deep vein thrombosis
- Decreased range of motion and strength of the gastroc-soleus muscles
- Complex regional pain syndrome (CRPS) (see Table 3-4)

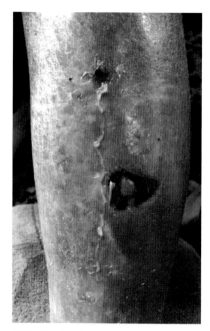

FIGURE 3-22. Secondary lymphedema after orthopedic surgery.

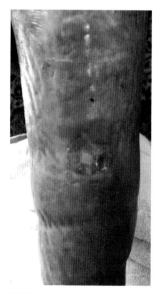

FIGURE 3-23. Lower extremity after 2 weeks of multi-layer compression and exercise.

Clinical presentation
- Ipsilateral edema of the extremity, usually distal to the most proximal incisional area
- May include erythema, pruritis, pain, changes in skin color, increased skin temperature

TABLE 3-4.   Stages and symptoms of Complex Regional Pain Syndrome

1. Continuing pain, disproportionate to the inciting event	
2. At least one symptom in three of the following categories:	a. Sensory: hyperesthesia (an abnormal increase in sensitivity) and/or allodynia (pain caused by usually non-painful stimuli)
	b. Vasomotor: skin color changes or temperature and/or skin color changes between the limbs
	c. Sudomotor/edema: edema (swelling) and/or sweating changes and/or sweating differences between the limbs
	d. Motor/trophic: decreased range of motion and/or motor dysfunction (weakness, tremor, muscular spasm (dystonia)) and/or trophic changes (changes to the hair and/or nail and/or skin on the limb)
3. At least one sign in two of the following categories:	a. Sensory: hyperalgesia (to pinprick) and/or allodynia [to light touch and/or deep somatic (physical) pressure and/or joint movement]
	b. Vasomotor: temperature differences between the limbs and/or skin color changes and/or skin color changes between the limbs
	c. Sudomotor/edema: edema and/or sweating changes and/or sweating differences between the limbs
	d. Motor/trophic: decreased range of motion and/or motor dysfunction (i.e. weakness, tremor, or muscle spasm) and/or trophic changes (hair and/or nail and/or skin changes)
4. No other diagnosis explaining the symptoms and signs	

(Data from Complex Regional Pain Syndrome. https://www.blbchronicpain.co.uk/news/what-are-the-crps-budapest-criteria/)

Medical management
- Determine the exact cause of the occlusion
- Perform vascular screening for arterial disease
- Apply compression with short-stretch bandages or intermittent compression pump (in case of vascular surgery)[16]
- Refer to physical therapy for range of motion and strengthening exercise of involved extremity
- Refer to lymphedema specialist for manual lymphatic drainage[23]

Wound management
- Standard wound care in the case of skin breakdown or traumatic wounds that occur on the edematous extremity

KLIPPEL TRENAUNAY WEBER SYNDROME

Figures 3-24 through 3-27

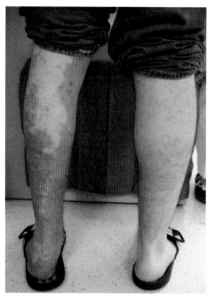

FIGURE 3-24. Port wine staining on the posterior lower extremities.

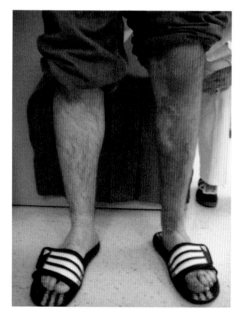

FIGURE 3-25. Port wine staining on the anterior lower extremities. Note the leg length discrepancy on the left leg, as well as the muscle atrophy that makes edema less evident. Palpation, testing for pitting, and measurements are needed to confirm the presence of edema.

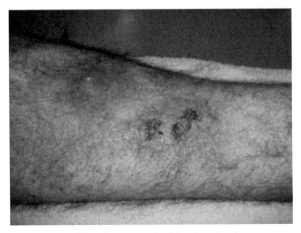

FIGURE 3-26. Wounds as a result of the chronic edema.

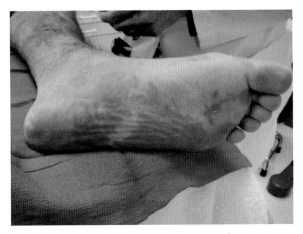

FIGURE 3-27. Port wine staining on the plantar foot.

Pathophysiology
- A rare congenital disorder with varicosities and/or venous malformation, capillary malformation, and boney and/or soft tissue malformation of the limbs[24]
- May include absence of the femoral and iliac venous systems

Clinical presentation
- Port wine staining of a large portion of the body
- Lower extremity size discrepancy in both girth and length with resulting leg length discrepancy
- Varicosities
- Wounds in the gaiter area, consistent with CVI
- Pitting edema with possible obscuring of pulses

Medical management
- Referral to a vascular surgeon for possible surgical reconstruction of the venous system
- Referral to an orthotist for shoe inserts, in the case of leg length discrepancy
- Laser and/or ablative therapy for capillary malformation

Wound management
- Debridement of necrotic tissue
- Appropriate primary dressings depending on drainage and signs of microbes
- Compression therapy

SUMMARY

Venous wounds respond well when treated appropriately; however, venous wounds that fail to heal, or decrease significantly in size, after 6 weeks of evidence-based care as described above should have further diagnostic tests to rule out those etiologies that may *appear* as venous wounds but are indeed caused by other pathologies.[25] (See Table 3-5.) Continuation of compression with some type of garment, device, or intermittent compression pump is imperative in order to prevent recurrence of the venous wounds. Patients need to be instructed to replace garments every 3–6 months, or whenever they lose their integrity and no longer manage the edema effectively.[11]

TABLE 3-5.   Wounds that may appear to be venous wounds but are caused by other pathologies

Malignancies
Vasculitis
Polyarteritis nodosum
Vasculopathy
Pyoderma gangrenosum
Mycobacterial or fungal infections
Necrobiosis lipoidica diabeticum
Systemic lupus erythematosus wounds
Cryoglobulinemia

REFERENCES

1. Villeco JP. Edema: A silent but important factor. *Journal of Hand Therapy.* 2012;25(2): 153-162.
2. Eberhardt RT, Raffetto JD. Chronic venous insufficiency. *Circulation.* 2005;111: 2398-23409.
3. O'Donnell TF, Passman MA, Marston WA, Ennis WJ, Dalsing M, Kisner RL, et al. Management of venous leg ulcers: Clinical practice guidelines of the Society for Vascular Surgery® and the American Venous Forum. *Journal of Vascular Surgery.* 2014;60:3S-59S.
4. Woelfel S, Ochoa C, Rowe VL. Vascular wounds. In Hamm RL, ed. *Text and Atlas of Wound Diagnosis and Treatment.* 2nd ed. New York: McGraw-Hill Education. 2019;101-143.
5. Alavi A, Hafner J, Dutz JP, Mayer D, Sibbald RG, Criado PR, et al. Atrophie Blanche: Is it associated with venous disease or livedoid vasculopathy? *Advances in Skin and Wound Care.* 2014;27(11):518-524.
6. Rai R. Standard guidelines for the management of venous leg ulcer. *Indian Dermatology Online Journal.* 2014;5(3):408-411. doi:10.4103/2229-5178.137830. Accessed September 21, 2019.

7. Hettrick H. The science of compression therapy for chronic venous insufficiency edema. *The Journal of the American College of certified Wound Specialists.* 2009;1(1):20-24.

8. White J, Ivins N, Wilkes A, Carolan-Rees G, Harding KG. Non-contact low-frequency ultrasound therapy compared with UK standard of care for venous leg ulcers: a single-centre, assessor-blinded, randomized controlled trial. *International Wound Journal.* 2016;13(5):833-42.

9. Gibbons GW, Orgill DP, Serena TE, Novoung A, O.Connell JB, Li WW, et al. A prospective, randomized, controlled trial comparing the effects of noncontact, low-frequency ultrasound to standard care in healing venous leg ulcers. *Ostomy Wound Management.* 2015;61(1):16-29.

10. Trayes KP, Studdiford JS, Pickle S, Tully AS. Edema: Diagnosis and management. American Academy of Family Physicians. Available at https://lipedemaproject.org/wp-content/uploads/2016/02/2013_Trayes_Edema-Diagnosis-and-Management.pdf. Accessed September 23, 2019.

11. Perdomo M, Hamm RL. Lymphedema. In Hamm RL ed. *Text and Atlas of Wound Diagnosis and Treatment.* 2nd ed. New York: McGraw-Hill Education. 2019;145-169.

12. Ratchford EV, Evans NS. Approach to lower extremity edema. *Current Treatment Options in Cardiovascular Medicine.* 2017;19(3):16.

13. Cormier JN, Rourke L, Crosby M, Chang D, Armer J. The surgical treatment of lymphedema: A systematic review of the contemporary literature (2004-2010). *Annals of Surgical Oncology.* 2012;19(2):642-651.

14. Granzow JW, Soderberg JM, Kaji AH, Dauphine C. An effective system of surgical treatment of lymphedema. *Annals of Surgical Oncology.* 2014;21(4):1189-1194.

15. Gallagher K, Marulanda K, Gray S. Surgical intervention for lymphedema. *Surgical Oncology Clinics of North America.* 2018;27(1):195-215.

16. Shavit E, Alavi A, Wollina U. Lipedema – is not lymphedema: A review of current literature. *International Wound Journal.* 2018;15(6):921-928.

17. Child AH, Gordon KD, Sharpe P, Brice G, Ostergaard P, Jeffery S, Mortimer PS. Lipedema: An inherited condition. *American Journal of Medical Genetics Part A.* 2010;152A:970-976 .

18. Dadras M, Mallinger PJ, Corterier CC, Dadras M, Theodosiadi S, Ghods M. Liposuction in the treatment of lipedema: A longitudinal study. *Archives of Plastic Surgery.* 2017;44(4):324-331.

19. El Tal AK, Tannous Z. Cutaneous vascular disorders associated with internal malignancy. *Dermatologic Clinics.* 2008;26(1):45-57.

20. Pawlaczyk K, Gabriel M, Urbanek T, Dzieciuchowicz L, Krasinski A, Gabriel Z, et al. Effects of intermittent pneumatic compression on reduction of postoperative lower extremity edema and normalization of foot microcirculation flow in patients undergoing arterial revascularization. *Medical Science Monitor.* 2015;21:3986-3992.

21. AbuRahma AF, Woodruff BA, Lucente FC. Edema after femoropopliteal bypass surgery: Lymphatic and venous theories of causation. *Journal of Vascular Surgery.* 1990;11(3):461-467.

22. Shieh AK, Lum AC, Singh AK, Pereira GC. External iliac vein compression secondary to osteolysis-induced hematoma in total hip arthroplasty. *Arthroplasty Today.* 2019;5(3):279-283.

23. Ebert JR, Joss B, Jardine B, Wood DJ. Randomized trial investigating the efficacy of manual lymphatic drainage to improve early outcome after total knee arthroplasty. *Archives of Physical Medicine and Rehabilitation.* 2013;94(11):2103-2111.

24. Shahbahrami K, Resnikoff M, Shah AY, Lydon RP, Lazar A, Cavallo G. Chronic lower extremity wounds in a patient with Klippel Trenaunay syndrome. *Journal of Vascular Surgery Cases and Innovative Techniques.* 2019;5(1):45-48.

25. Eberhardt RT, Raffetp JD. Chronic venous insufficiency. *Circulation.* 2005;111:2398-2409.

4

Pressure Injury/Ulcers

INTRODUCTION

Pressure injury/ulcers (PI/PUs) are a result of prolonged direct pressure, shear, or friction forces that injure soft tissue between the skin and underlying bony prominences. The sacrum/coccyx, heels, and greater trochanters are the anatomical areas most vulnerable to tissue injury; however, PUs can also occur on the occiput, ear, spine, scapula, acromion process, elbow, medial and lateral femoral condyles, patella, malleoli, and metatarsals—anywhere that there is little or no soft tissue over the bony prominence to dissipate the external and internal mechanical forces. The area most at risk depends upon the individual's body build. Therefore, any treatment plan for prevention and/or treatment has to be very patient-specific. The global strategies for prevention are repositioning, mobilization, frequent skin assessments, skin protection, moisture management, adequate nutrition, and avoidance of shear and friction during functional activities. And of paramount importance is finding the source of the mechanical pressure, which is not always what it appears to be initially. For example, a PU on the lateral hip may appear to be from lying on one side too long; however, it could also occur from sitting in a wheelchair that is too narrow.[1] The root-cause analysis of a PU, especially a deeper one, is determined by what the patient was doing, the surface upon which the patient was sitting/lying, and other risk factors, 48 hours prior to admission to a facility.[2]

Moisture per se is no longer considered a cause of pressure injury; however, exposure to urinary or fecal incontinence, wound drainage, or perspiration causes the skin to break down, therefore making it easier for bacteria to penetrate the skin. Moisture also changes the pH of the skin. Both of these consequences can increase the risk for a PU to develop and affect the healing potential. Other conditions that can affect the ability of the tissue to withstand pressure and shear are the microclimate, nutrition, perfusion, co-morbidities (e.g. diabetes, cardiac disease), and condition of the soft tissue (e.g. presence of scarring from previous wound healing, emaciation). All of these factors are to be considered when evaluating a patient with a PU, in addition to performing a vascular assessment of any lower extremity that may have compromised healing due to arterial insufficiency.

Treatment of the wound itself includes debridement of necrotic tissue and biofilm (either sharp, surgical, or enzymatic depending on the amount of tissue to be removed and the patient medical status), treatment of any infection, moist wound healing, and adjunct therapies when appropriate (e.g. electrical stimulation, pulsed lavage with suction, ultraviolet C, negative pressure wound therapy).

The National Pressure Injury Advisory Panel (NPIAP) has developed six classifi-cations of PUs based on the depth of tissue damage,[3] and although the Panel uses the term pressure injury,[4] Center for Medicare & Medicaid Services (CMS) still refers to them as PUs in the ICD-10 coding.[4] NPIAP also describes other skin disorders frequently documented as PUs that are indeed not PUs, e.g. device-related tissue injury, dermatitis, excoriation, and skin tears. Each pressure ulcer/injury stage is defined and illustrated in this chapter, as well as skin damage that is not considered a PU. Because pathophysiology and medical treatment for all PUs are similar, only wound management will be addressed for each of the stages.

* For this discussion, pressure injury shall refer to tissue damage with the skin intact, and pressure ulcer shall refer to tissue damage with loss of dermal tissue.

STAGE 1 PRESSURE INJURY: NON-BLANCHABLE ERYTHEMA OF INTACT SKIN

Figures 4-1 through 4-4

Intact skin with a localized area of non-blanchable erythema, which may appear differently in darkly pigmented skin. Presence of blanchable erythema or changes in sensation, temperature, or firmness may precede visual changes. Color changes do not include purple or maroon discoloration; these may indicate Deep Tissue Pressure Injury.

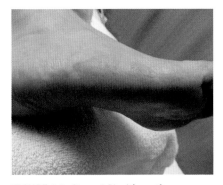

FIGURE 4-1. Stage 1 PI with erythema.

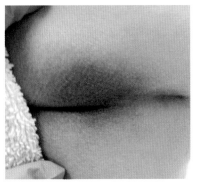

FIGURE 4-2. Stage 1 PI with change in skin texture.

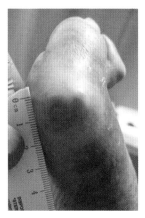

FIGURE 4-3. **Stage 1 PI on the heel.**

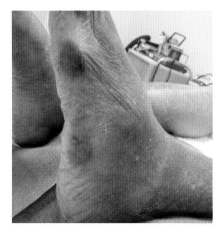

FIGURE 4-4. **Stage 1 PI on the lateral foot.**

Wound management
- Reposition frequently or off-load the affected area
- Cover with silicone-backed foam dressing to prevent further tissue damage.
- Refer to a registered dietician to optimize hydration and nutrition[5]
- Expect healing in 2–3 days with no scarring

STAGE 2 PRESSURE INJURY: PARTIAL-THICKNESS SKIN LOSS WITH EXPOSED DERMIS

Figures 4-5 through 4-9

The wound bed is viable, pink or red, moist, and may also present as an intact or ruptured serum-filled blister. Adipose (fat) is not visible and deeper tissues are not visible. Granulation tissue, slough, and eschar are not present. These injuries commonly result from adverse microclimate and shear in the skin over the pelvis and shear in the heel. This stage should not be used to describe moisture associated skin damage (MASD) including incontinence associated dermatitis (IAD), intertriginous dermatitis (ITD), medical adhesive-related skin injury (MARSI), or traumatic wounds (skin tears, burns, abrasions).

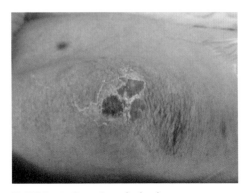

FIGURE 4-5. Stage 2 on the heel.

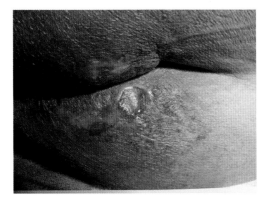

FIGURE 4-6. Stage 2 pressure ulcer on the right buttock.

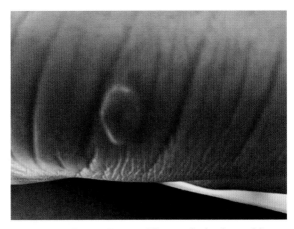

FIGURE 4-7. Stage 2 Pressure Ulcer on the heel; note blister is filled with clear fluid.

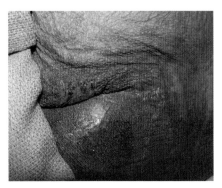

FIGURE 4-8. Stage 2 Pressure Ulcer on the buttocks.

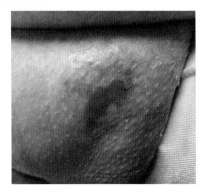

FIGURE 4-9. Stage 2 Pressure Ulcer on the buttocks with evidence of re-epithelialization at the edges.

Wound management
- Cleanse wound with a non-cytotoxic wound cleanser or tap water and cover with a protective dressing (e.g. silicone-backed foam with adhesive edges or thin hydrocolloid)[6]
- Apply electrical stimulation to facilitate epithelial migration across the wound surface[7,8,9]
- Reposition frequently or off-load the affected area with an appropriate support device
- Refer to a registered dietician to optimize hydration and nutrition[10,11,12]
- Expect healing in approximately 23 days, depending on the ulcer size, with little or no scarring;[13] only re-epithelialization is required for closure

STAGE 3: FULL THICKNESS TISSUE LOSS

Figures 4-10 through 4-14

Full-thickness loss of skin, in which adipose (fat) is visible in the ulcer; granulation tissue and epibole (rolled wound edges) are often present. Slough and/or eschar may be visible. The depth of tissue damage varies by anatomical location; areas of significant adiposity can develop deep wounds. Undermining and tunneling may occur. Fascia, muscle, tendon, ligament, cartilage, and/or bone are not exposed. If slough or eschar obscures the extent of tissue loss, this is an Unstageable Pressure Injury.

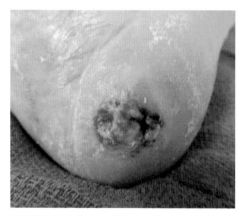

FIGURE 4-10. Stage 3 Pressure Ulcer on the heel.

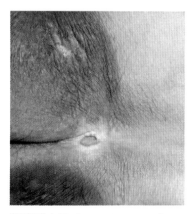

FIGURE 4-11. Stage 3 Pressure Ulcer on the coccyx (left buttock appears to have a Stage 2).

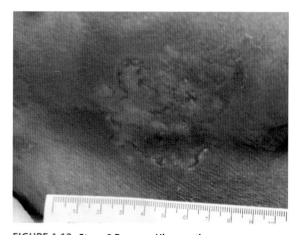

FIGURE 4-12. Stage 3 Pressure Ulcer on the sacrum.

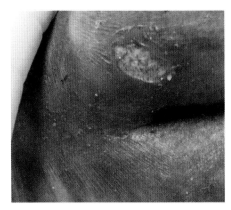

FIGURE 4-13. Stage 3 Pressure Ulcer on the right buttock; diffuse Stage 2 Pressure Ulcers on the sacrum and in the crease of the buttocks, often referred to as "kissing ulcers" This would need to be differentiated from moisture-associated skin damage, based on moisture exposure versus mechanical forces.

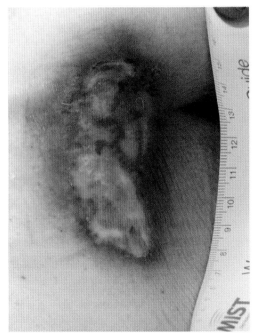

FIGURE 4-14. Stage 3 pressure ulcer in the proliferative phase of healing.

> **Diagnostic Clue:** Figure 4-14 is classified as a Stage 3 in the proliferative phase of healing, and when fully re-epithelialized, would be a Stage 3 in the remodeling phase. PUs are not staged backwards!

Wound management
- Debride necrotic tissue and apply an absorbent or hydrating dressing (depending on the amount of exudate) to maintain moisture balance[14]; fill any undermining to avoid leaving a dead space where exudate can accumulate and create an environment for bacterial growth.

- Treat any critical colonization present with topical antimicrobial dressings or with ultraviolet C; administer systemic antibiotics only if signs of periwound infection are present[15]
- Apply electrical stimulation to facilitate granulation formation and re-epithelialization[16,17]
- Apply advanced dressings (e.g. collagen,[18] human amniotic epithelial cells,[19] cellular/tissue dressings) for larger or hard-to-heal wounds
- Reposition frequently or off-load the affected area; in the case of multiple wounds, provide a special support surface for bed or wheelchair[20]
- Keep the head of the bed flat or below 30° unless otherwise contraindicated (e.g. if the patient has a gastrointestinal feeding tube)
- Refer to a registered dietician to optimize hydration and nutrition[21,22]

STAGE 4: FULL THICKNESS SKIN AND TISSUE LOSS

Figures 4-15 through 4-22

Full-thickness skin and tissue loss with exposed or directly palpable fascia, muscle, tendon, ligament, cartilage or bone in the ulcer. Slough and/or eschar may be visible. Epibole (rolled edges), undermining and/or tunneling often occur. Depth varies by anatomical location. If slough or eschar obscures the extent of tissue loss, this is an Unstageable Pressure Injury.

Stage 4 ulcers can extend into muscle and/or supporting structures (e.g. fascia, tendon, or joint capsule), making osteomyelitis or osteitis likely to occur. Exposed bone/muscle is visible or directly palpable.

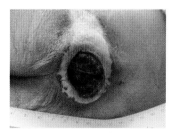

FIGURE 4-15. Stage 4 Pressure Ulcer on the sacrum.

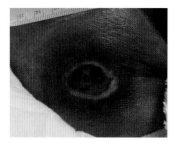

FIGURE 4-16. Stage 4 Pressure Ulcer with epibole at the edges.

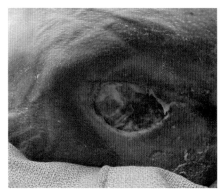

FIGURE 4-17. Stage 4 Pressure Ulcer with exposed muscle and bone.

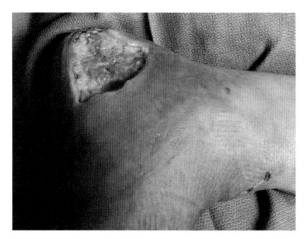

FIGURE 4-18. Stage 4 Pressure Ulcer on the heel; dark shadow on the anterior edge is an indication of undermining.

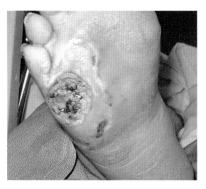

FIGURE 4-19. Stage 4 Pressure Ulcer with exposed bone palpable with a metal instrument.

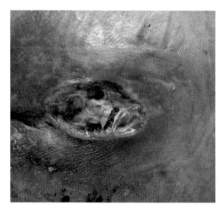

FIGURE 4-20. Stage 4 Pressure Ulcer with non-viable fascia.

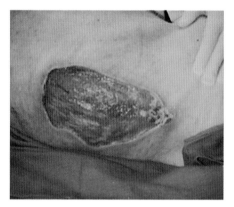

FIGURE 4-21. Stage 4 Pressure Ulcer on the dorsal trunk with exposed spinal process at the distal aspect.

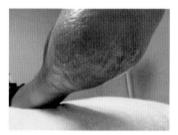

FIGURE 4-22. Stage 4 healed and in the remodeling phase.

Wound management
- Sharp or surgical debridement of all necrotic tissue
- Pulsed lavage with suction[23]
- Negative pressure wound therapy

- Assessment for osteomyelitis if bone is exposed[4,24]
- Pressure-relieving support surface (low-air loss, alternating pressure, or air fluidized)
- Maintenance of the head of the bed flat or below 30° unless otherwise contraindicated
- Referral to a registered dietician to optimize hydration and nutrition
- Referral to a plastic surgeon for possible flap coverage

DEEP TISSUE PRESSURE INJURY: PERSISTENT NON-BLANCHABLE DEEP RED, MAROON, OR PURPLE DISCOLORATION

Figures 4-23 through 4-27

Intact or non-intact skin with localized area of persistent non-blanchable deep red, maroon, or purple discoloration or epidermal separation revealing a dark wound bed or blood filled blister. Pain and temperature change often precede skin color changes. Discoloration may appear differently in darkly pigmented skin. This injury results from intense and/or prolonged pressure and shear forces at the bone-muscle interface. The wound may evolve rapidly to reveal the actual extent of tissue injury, or may resolve without tissue loss. If necrotic tissue, subcutaneous tissue, granulation tissue, fascia, muscle or other underlying structures are visible, this indicates a full thickness pressure injury (Unstageable, Stage 3, or Stage 4). Do not use DTPI to describe vascular, traumatic, neuropathic, or dermatologic conditions.

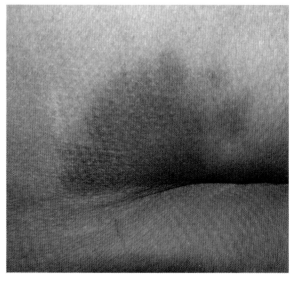

FIGURE 4-23. DTPI on the right sacrum.

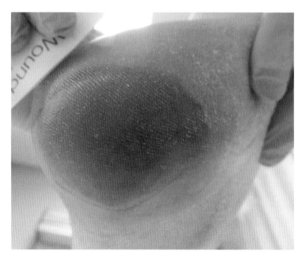

FIGURE 4-24. DTPI on the heel with blood-filled blister.

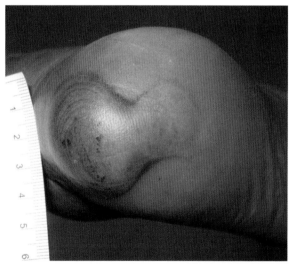

FIGURE 4-25. DTPI progressing toward an Unstageable PI.

Diagnostic Clue: Blisters filled with serous fluid are from friction that produces an inflammatory response between the epidermis and dermis, and are thus partial thickness Stage 2 PUs. Blisters filled with blood are from capillary disruption and bleeding in the deeper soft tissue, and are thus Deep Tissue Pressure Injuries.

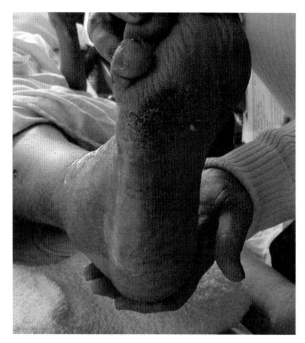

FIGURE 4-26. DPTI on the heel.

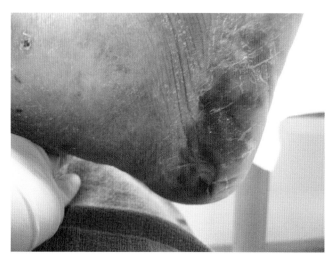

FIGURE 4-27. DTPI progressing toward an Unstageable PI.

Wound management
- Reposition frequently off the affected area
- Place on a pressure-relieving support surface
- Apply a protective silicone-backed dressing[25]
- Treat with non-contact low-frequency ultrasound[26]

- Optimize hydration and nutrition
- Observe the evolution of the DTPI and document changes in stage if indicated by the appearance or the depth of the injured tissue (DTPI may become Unstageable, Stage 3, or Stage 4 PUs)

UNSTAGEABLE PRESSURE INJURY: OBSCURED FULL-THICKNESS SKIN AND TISSUE LOSS

Figures 4-28 through 4-34

Full-thickness skin and tissue loss in which the extent of tissue damage within the ulcer cannot be confirmed because it is obscured by slough or eschar. If slough or eschar is removed, a Stage 3 or Stage 4 pressure injury will be revealed. Stable eschar (i.e. dry, adherent, and intact without erythema or fluctuance) on the heel or ischemic limb should not be softened or removed.

Wound management—stable eschar
- Clean edges and debride only loose, unattached, non-viable tissue
- Off-load with the appropriate device or support surface
- Periodically trim the loose eschar edge as the epithelium migrates under the eschar to prevent inadvertent pulling away from the skin
- Do not moisten or soften by soaking or applying a wet dressing
- Debride all of the eschar if erythema, fluctuance, or other signs of infection appear

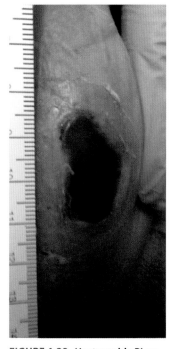

FIGURE 4-28. Unstageable PI on the heel with stable eschar.

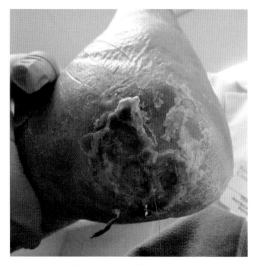

FIGURE 4-29. Unstageable PI with loose necrotic tissue at the edges.

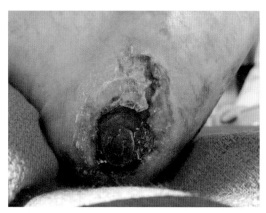

FIGURE 4-30. Unstageable PI with detached eschar and periwound signs of infection; loose necrotic tissue can be debrided to further evaluate eschar status.

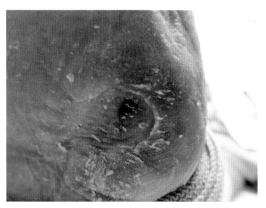

FIGURE 4-31. Unstageable PI with stable eschar after removal of detached necrotic tissue.

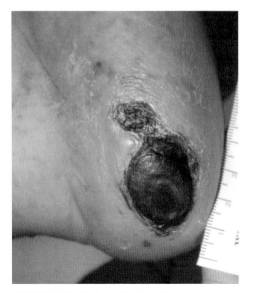

FIGURE 4-32. Unstageable PI stable eschar.

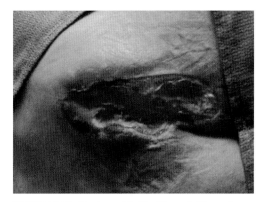

FIGURE 4-33. Unstageable PI with unstable eschar.

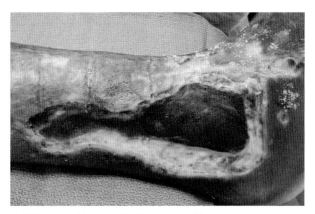

FIGURE 4-34. Unstageable PI with unstable eschar.

Wound management—unstable eschar
- Debride the non-viable tissue; stage appropriately
- Treat according to guidelines for the appropriate stage

MEDICAL-DEVICE RELATED PRESSURE INJURY

Figures 4-35 through 4-39

Medical device-related pressure injuries result from the use of devices designed and applied for diagnostic or therapeutic purposes. The resultant pressure injury generally conforms to the pattern or shape of the device. The injury should be staged using the staging system (along with the causative device).[4]

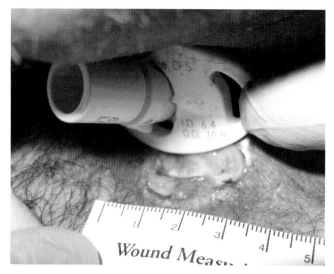

FIGURE 4-35. Stage 3 PI under an endotracheal tube.

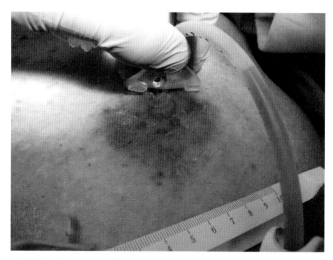

FIGURE 4-36. Stage 2 PI under a PEG collar with excoriation from gastric fluid leakage.

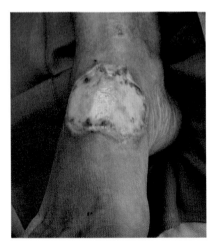

FIGURE 4-37. Unstageable PI due to compression wrap after surgery for a kidney transplant.

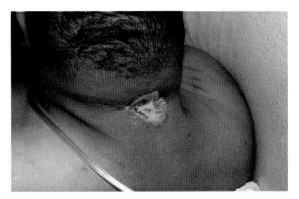

FIGURE 4-38. Necrosis of posterior neck from tape used to anchor an ET tube; unable to stage from photograph.
Used with permission from Aimee Garcia.

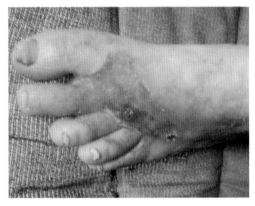

FIGURE 4-39. Stage 3 PI in the proliferative phase; from a cast applied too tightly.

Wound management
- Cleanse the wound, debride necrotic tissue, and dress appropriately
- Either change the position of the device, place a thick foam dressing between the skin and the device, or eliminate the use of the device
- Check the area frequently if the device needs to remain in place

> **Diagnostic Clue:** Any complaint of pain under a medical device (e.g. cast, brace, tube, compression wrap) is addressed by removal of the device and inspection of the skin unless the physician has written specific orders not to remove the device. In that case, the physician should be informed of the patient's complaint of pain under the device. Undetected pressure injuries under causative devices will only worsen with time if the pressure is not relieved. Treating the complaint with pain medication without determining the cause of the pain is not adequate care.

MUCOSAL MEMBRANE PRESSURE INJURY

Mucosal membrane pressure injury is found on mucous membranes with a history of a medical device in use at the location of the injury. Due to the anatomy of the tissue, these injuries cannot be staged.

Wound management
- Cleanse the wound with normal saline and position the medical device away from the injury
- Anchor the device/tube if possible so that it does not create friction on the affected area
- Change the position of the tube (e.g. an NG tube) frequently so that pressure is not maintained in one area
- Involve all of the disciplines (e.g. nursing, respiratory, dietary, therapy services) in repositioning strategies

MOISTURE-ASSOCIATED SKIN DAMAGE

Figures 4-40 through 4-45

Moisture-associated skin damage is inflammation and erosion of the skin caused by prolonged exposure to moisture from wound drainage, fecal or urinary incontinence, mucus or saliva, perspiration, peristomal drainage, or dressings that are too wet.[27] The moisture damages the outer layer of the epidermis thus making the skin more susceptible to friction and shear. The damaged skin can also become a portal for bacteria and thereby increase the risk for infection.[25] When moisture-associated skin damage occurs in the skin folds, e.g. under the pannus, it is termed *intertriginous dermatitis*.

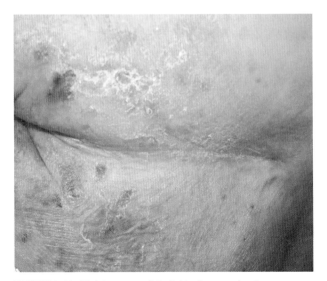

FIGURE 4-40. Moisture-associated skin damage due to
incontinence.

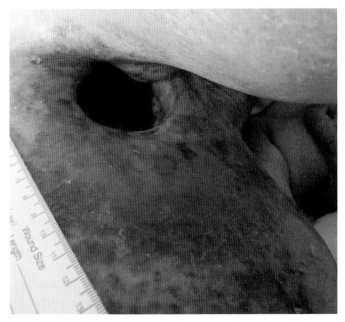

FIGURE 4-41. Moisture-associated skin damage due to wound drainage.

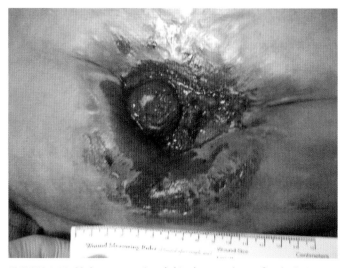

FIGURE 4-42. Moisture-associated skin damage due to fistula drainage.

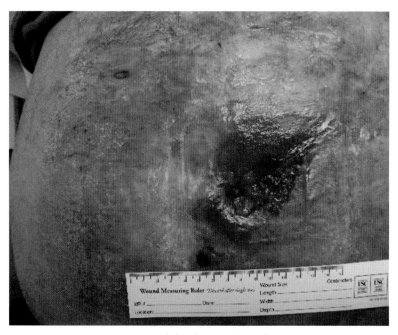

FIGURE 4-43. Moisture-associated skin damage due to fistula drainage.

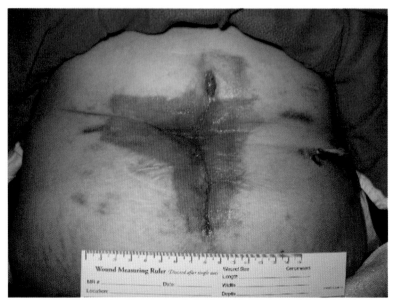

FIGURE 4-44. Medical adhesive-related skin injury (MARSI).

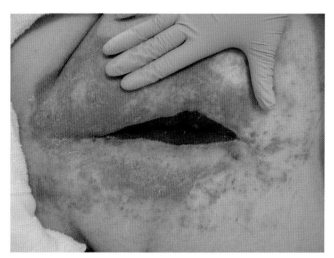

FIGURE 4-45. MARSI under the film used with negative pressure wound therapy.

Diagnostic Clue: An indication that skin damage is due to a medical adhesive is the distinct line of erythema that parallels the shape of the adhesive device (Figures 4-44 and 4-45).

TERMINAL ULCERS

Figures 4-46 through 4-48

End-of-life skin changes that appear as pressure injuries have been termed Kennedy terminal ulcer, Skin Changes at Life's End (SCALE), and Trombley-Brennan terminal

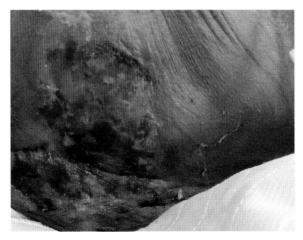

FIGURE 4-46. Terminal ulcer on the sacrum.

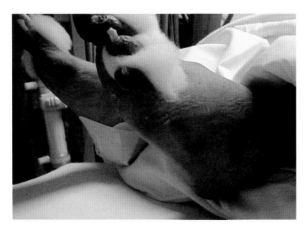

FIGURE 4-47. Lamb's wool placed between the toes to prevent maceration due to SCALE.

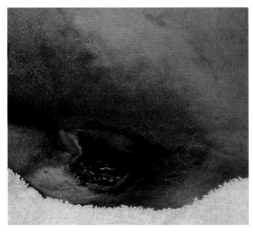

FIGURE 4-48. Terminal ulcer on the sacrum.

tissue injury.[28] A consensus statement issued in 2010 defined terminal ulcers as the following: "Physiological changes that occur as a result of the dying process may affect the skin and soft tissues and may manifest as observable (objective) changes in skin color, turgor, or integrity or as subjective symptoms such as localized pain. These changes can be unavoidable and may occur even with the application of appropriate interventions that meet or exceed the standard of care (sic for the prevention of pressure ulcers).[29] Hypoperfusion is thought to be a critical contributing factor to the formation of these tissue injuries,[30] along with the failure of two or more organs.[27] Clinical signs may include red, yellow, or black bilateral ulcers on the sacrum or coccyx;[31] mottled discoloration and skin necrosis that may occur within 6–8 hours, a shorter time period than is usual for full-thickness or Deep Tissue Pressure Injuries.[27] In addition to addressing underlying co-morbidities, the SCALE consensus recommended the 5 Ps for determining appropriate intervention strategies:

• Prevention if at all possible, realizing that some are considered unavoidable
• Prescription (if it is possible for healing to occur with appropriate treatment)
• Preservation (maintenance without deterioration)
• Palliation (interventions based on patient comfort and family solace)
• Preference (for patient desires)[28]

WOUNDS MISTAKEN FOR PRESSURE INJURIES

Wounds frequently seen upon admission to a facility that should not be designated as pressure injuries include skin tears, bruises from trauma, subcutaneous bleeds from medication, diabetic foot ulcers, abscesses, infections, burns, and rarely but importantly malignancies.[1] Misdiagnosis can lead to ineffective treatment, miscoding that affects hospital reimbursement, and poor patient outcomes, whereas correct diagnosis leads to appropriate treatment, faster healing, and less cost for care.

REFERENCES

1. Garcia A, Sprigle S. Pressure injuries and ulcers. In Hamm R, ed. *Text and Atlas of Wound Diagnosis and Treatmen.*, 2nd ed. New York: McGraw Hill Education. 2019;171-198.
2. Black J. Pressure Ulcer Prevention: More Than Turning and Beds. Available at https://www.nyspfp.org/Materials/Black_Pressure_Ulcer_Presentation_6_5_13.pdf. Accessed November 9, 2019.
3. National Pressure Ulcer Advisory Panel. NPUAP Pressure Injury Stages. Available at https://cdn.ymaws.com/npuap.site-ym.com/resource/resmgr/npuap_pressure_injury_stages.pdf. Accessed October 21,2019.
4. Edsberg LE, Black JM, Goldberg M, McNichol L, Moore L, Sieggreen M. Revised National Pressure Ulcer Advisory Panel Pressure Injury Staging System. *Journal of Wound, Ostomy, and Continence Nursing.* 2016;43(6):585-597.
5. National Pressure Ulcer Advisory Panel, European Pressure Ulcer Advisory Panel and Pan Pacific Pressure Injury Alliance. Prevention and Treatment of Pressure Ulcers: Nutrition – an extract from the Clinical Practice Guideline. Emily Haesler (Ed.). Cambridge Media: Osborne Park, Western Australia; 2014.
6. Payne WG, Posnett J, Alvarez O, Brown-Etris M, Jameson G, Wolcott R, et al. A prospective, randomized clinical trial to assess the cost-effectiveness of a modern foam dressing versus a traditional saline gauze dressing in the treatment of stage II pressure ulcers. *Ostomy Wound Manage.* 2009;55(2):50-55.

7. Polak A, Kloth LC, Blaszczak E, Taradaj J, Nawrat-Szoltysik A, Walczak A, et al. Evaluation of the healing progress of pressure ulcers treated with cathodal high-voltage monophasic pulsed current: Results of a prospective, double-blind, randomized clinical trial. *Advances in Skin and Wound Care.* 2016;29(10):447-459.
8. Bora Karsli P, Gurcay E, Karaahmet OZ, Cakci A. High-voltage electrical stimulation versus ultrasound in the treatment of pressure ulcers. *Advances in Skin and Wound Care.* 2017;30(12):565-570.
9. Girgis B, Duarte JA. High voltage monophasic pulsed current (HVMPC) for stage II-IV pressure ulcer healing. A systematic review and meta-analysis. *Journal of Tissue Viability.* 2018;27(4):274-284.
10. National Pressure Ulcer Advisory Panel, European Pressure Ulcer Advisory Panel and Pan Pacific Pressure Injury Alliance. Prevention and Treatment of Pressure Ulcers: Nutrition – an extract from the Clinical Practice Guideline. Emily Haesler, ed. Cambridge Media: Osborne Park, Western Australia; 2014.
11. Cereda E, Gini A, Pedrolli C, Vanotti A. Disease-specific, versus standard, nutritional support for the treatment of pressure ulcers in institutionalized older adults: a randomized control trial. *Journal of the American Geriatric Society.* 2009;57(8):1395-1402.
12. Cereda E, Klersy C, Serioli M, Crespi A, D'Andrea F. A nutritional formula enriched with arginine, zinc, and antioxidants for the healing of pressure ulcers: A randomized trial. *Annals of Internal Medicine.* 2015;162(3):167-174.
13. Palese A, Luisa S, Ilenia P, Laquintana D, Stinco G, Di Giulio P, PARI-ETLD Group. What is the healing time of Stage II pressure ulcers? Findings from a secondary analysis. *Advances in Skin and Wound Care.* 2015;28(2):69-75.
14. Souliotis K, Kalemikerakis I, Saridi M, Papageorgiou M, Kalokerinou A. A cost and clinical effectiveness analysis among moist wound healing dressings versus traditional methods in home care patients with pressure ulcers. *Wound Repair and Regeneration.* 2016;24(3):596-601.
15. Tedeschi S, Negosanti L, Sgarzani R, Trapani F, Pignanelli S, Battilana M, et al. Superficial swab versus deep-tissue biopsy for the microbiological diagnosis of local infection in advanced-stage pressure ulcers of spinal-cord-injured patients: A prospective study. *Clinical Microbiology and Infection.* 2017;23:943-947.
16. Houghton PE, Campbell KE, Fraser CH, Harris C, Keast DH, Potter PJ, et al. Electrical stimulation therapy increases rate of healing of pressure ulcers in community-dwelling people with spinal cord injury. *Archives of Physical Medicine and Rehabilitation.* 2010;91(5):669-678.
17. Polak A, Kloth LC, Paczula M, Nawrat-Szoltysik A, Kucio E, Manasar A, et al. Pressure injuries treated with anodal and cathodal high-voltage electrical stimulation: the effect on blood serum concentration of cytokines and growth factors in patients with neurological injuries. A randomized clinical study. *Wound Management and Prevention.* 2019;65(11):19-32.
18. Brown-Etris M, Milne CT, Hodde JP. An extracellular matrix graft (Oasis® wound matrix) for treating full-thickness pressure ulcers: A randomized clinical trial. *Journal of Tissue Viability.* 2019;28(1):21-26.
19. Zheng X, Jiang Z, Zhou A, Yu L, Quan M, Cheng H. Pathologic changes of wound tissue in rats with stage III pressure ulcers treated by transplantation of human amniotic epithelial cells. *International Journal of Clinical Experimental Pathology.* 2015;8(10):12284-91.
20. Makhsous M, Lin F, Knaus E, Zeigler M, Rowles DM, Gittler M, et al. Promote pressure ulcer healing in individuals with spinal cord injury using an individualized cyclic pressure-relief protocol. *Advances in Skin and Wound Care.* 2009;22(11):514-521.
21. Ohura T, Makajo T, Okada S, Omura K, Adachi K. Evaluation of effects of nutrition intervention on healing of pressure ulcers and nutritional states (randomized control trial). *Wound Repair and Regeneration.* 2011;19(3):330-336.

22. Neyens JCL, Cereda E, Meijer EP, Lindholm C, Schols JMGA. Arginine-enriched oral nutritional supplementation in the treatment of pressure ulcers: A literature review. *Wound Medicine.* 2017;16:45-51.
23. Ho CH, Bensitel T, Wang X, Bogie KM. Pulsatile lavage for the enhancement of pressure ulcer healing: a randomized controlled trial. *Physical Therapy.* 2012;92(1):38-48.
24. Brunel AS, Lamy B, Cyteval C, Perrochia H, Teot L, Masson R, et al. Diagnosing pelvic osteomyelitis beneath pressure ulcers in spinal cord injured patients: A prospective study. *Clin Microbiol Infect.* 2016;22:267.e1-267.e8. Available at http://cbc.doi.org/10.1016/j.cmi.2015.11.005.
25. Sullivan R. Use of a soft silicone foam dressing to change the trajectory of destruction associated with suspected deep tissue pressure ulcer. *MedSurg Nursing,* July-Aug. 2015, p. 237+. *Gale Academic Onefile.* Accessed November 10, 2019.
26. Honaker JS, Forston MR, Davis EA, Weisner MM, Morgan JA. Effect of non-contact low-frequency ultrasound on healing of suspected deep tissue injury: A retrospective analysis. *International Wound Journal.* 2012. Available at https://doi.org/10.1111/j.1742-481X.2012.00944.x. Accessed November 10, 2019.
27. Zulkowski K. Understanding moisture-associated skin damage, medical adhesive-related skin injuries, and skin tears. *Advances in Skin and Wound Care.* 2017;30(8):372-381.
28. Ayello EA, Levine JM, Langemo K, Kennedy-Evans KL, Brennan MR, Sibbald GR. Reexamining the literature on terminal ulcers, SCALE, skin failure, and unavoidable pressure injuries. *Advances in Skin and Wound Care.* 2019;32(3):109-121.
29. Sibbald GR, Krasner DL, Lutz JB, et al. Skin changes at life's end (SCALE): a preliminary consensus statement. *Advances in Skin and Wound Care.* 2010;23(5):225-236.
30. Yastrub DJ. Pressure or pathology: Distinguishing pressure ulcers from the Kennedy terminal ulcer. *JWOCN.* 2010;37:249-250.
31. Kennedy KL. The prevalence of pressure ulcers in an intermediate care facility. *Decubitus.* 1989;2(2):44-45.

5

Diabetic Foot Ulcers

Diabetic foot ulcers (DFUs) typically occur on the weight-bearing surface of the foot or the digits as a result of sensory neuropathy, bony abnormalities, and/or repeated mechanical forces (shear, friction, or direct pressure). Because patients with diabetes often present with other co-morbidities, including peripheral arterial disease (PAD), it is imperative to distinguish DFUs from other types of wounds in order to effectively diagnose and treat. A thorough vascular examination is a critical part of managing patients with DFUs, and if pedal pulses are diminished or absent, timely referral to a vascular specialist is warranted. If pedal pulses are present, DFUs can be treated with standard care as described below. However, even in the presence of palpable pedal pulses, referral to a vascular specialist should be considered for cases in which a wound fails to progress in a given period of time, or if the patient is at particularly high risk for amputation.

INTRODUCTION

> **Clinical Guideline:** Pulses are palpated with the ungloved finger directly over the dorsalis pedis and posterior tibial arteries, after removal of the patient's socks. If pulses are diminished and confirmed with a Doppler, note that a positive Doppler sound does not equate to normal blood flow. In this case, perfusion is reduced and referral to a vascular specialist for further testing is indicated.

Patients with hyperglycemia can have impaired healing of wounds due to any etiology (e.g. surgical incisions, venous, pressure, or trauma); however, these wounds are not termed diabetic wounds. Rather, they are classified according to their etiology, for example, a non-healing pressure ulcer on a patient with diabetes. This becomes important in coding for reimbursement. The American Diabetes Association guidelines for patients with diabetes recommend that hemoglobin A1c levels be 53 mmol/mol or <7%.[1] Hyperglycemia is known to impede wound healing by several mechanisms, (Table 5-1) as well as to increase the risk of infection; therefore, management of blood glucose levels is an integral component of treating any patient with diabetes who has a diabetic foot ulcer or non-healing wound.[2]

TABLE 5-1.   Impaired cellular function associated with diabetes

- Impaired neutrophil and macrophage function
- Excessive deposition of matrix proteins (collagen and fibronectin)
- Reaction of glucose with proteins to form advanced glycosylation end-products (AGEs)
- Decreased endothelial cell response to angiogenic stimuli
- Interference with cell communication and need for keratinocyte migration
- Decreased keratinocyte migration
- Failure of timely and rapid wound contraction
- Impaired endothelial function (nitric oxide)

Adapted with permission from Hamm RL: Text and Atlas of Wound Diagnosis and Treatment, 2nd ed. New York, NY: McGraw Hill; 2019.

Diagnostic Clue: The guidelines to help determine if infection is a result of poor glucose control or if the hyperglycemia is contributing to the infection are (1) if the patient's hemoglobin A1c is normal and blood glucose levels are high, the infection occurred first, resulting in hyperglycemia which is frequently the first sign indicating presence of infection; (2) if the hemoglobin A1c is high, the infection is more likely to be a result of the hyperglycemia. In the presence of hyperglycemia, the leukocytes will bind to the sugar molecules, thus making them ineffective for initiating an immune response to pathogens.

DIABETIC FOOT ULCERS

Figures 5-1 through 5-18

Pathophysiology

Prolonged hyperglycemia leads to glycosylation of multiple organ systems in the person with diabetes, resulting in intrinsic and extrinsic factors that lead to the foot's inability to withstand the mechanical stress of movement. The neuromuscular progression involves the following pathologies:

- Loss of protective sensation (defined as the inability to detect 10 grams of pressure on the plantar surface of the foot, as measured with the Semmes-Weinstein 5.07 monofilament)
- Loss of intrinsic foot muscles with an extrinsic muscle imbalance, causing tendons to pull abnormally on the joints and thereby resulting in bony deformities
- Increased mechanical pressure on the weight-bearing joints of the plantar foot with resulting pressure ischemia
- Hyperkeratosis of the skin over the bony abnormalities due to repeated friction
- Sublesional microhemorrhage and small areas of necrosis with repeated shearing, which in turn leads to larger subcutaneous tissue injury
- Localized inflammatory response with an increased skin temperature ≥4°F as compared to the same site on the contralateral foot[2]

- Increased risk of infection due to necrotic tissue and a dysfunctional immune response
- Dyshidrosis due to autonomic nervous dysfunction[2]

Clinical presentation

The University of Texas (UT) Wound Classification System is commonly used to classify DFUs based on the extent of tissue loss/depth of wound, and the presence of infection and/or ischemia. See Table 5-2 for a description of the UT Wound Classification System.[3] More recently, the Wound, Ischemia, and foot Infection (WIfI) classification

TABLE 5-2.   University of Texas Wound Classification System

		Grade			
		0	**1**	**2**	**3**
Stage	A	Pre or post ulcerative lesion completely epithelialized	Superficial wound, not involving tendon, capsule or bone	Wound penetrating to tendon or capsule	Wound penetrating to bone or joint
	B	Infection	Infection	Infection	Infection
	C	Ischemia	Ischemia	Ischemia	Ischemia
	D	Infection + Ischemia	Infection + Ischemia	Infection + Ischemia	Infection + Ischemia

Adapted with permission from Armstrong DG, Lavery LA, Harkless LB. Validation of a diabetic wound classification system. The contribution of depth, infection, and ischemia to risk of amputation, Diabetes Care. 1998 May;21(5): 855-859.

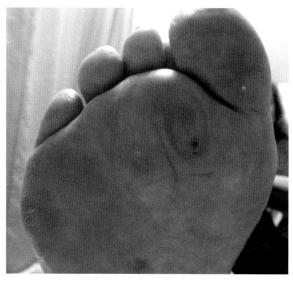

FIGURE 5-1. Foot at risk for ulceration with bony abnormality and preulcerative/hyperkeratotic plantar lesion (UT0).

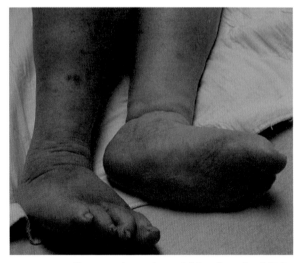

FIGURE 5-2. Charcot arthropathy, at risk for ulceration (UT0).

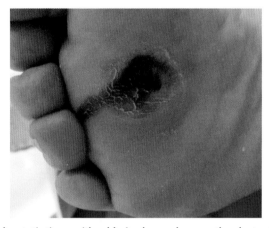

FIGURE 5-3. Hyperkeratotic tissue with sublesion hemorrhage on the plantar 3rd metatarsal head (before debridement) (UT1A).

(described in Chapter 2) has emerged as a valuable tool in evaluating patients with DFUs who are at risk for limb loss. The WIfI system is based on wound depth, infection, and perfusion status, and incorporates several other classification systems in order to comprehensively stratify amputation risk and aid in clinical decision making[4] (see Figure 2-1).

General characteristics of DFUs vary, and may include any of the following:

- Hyperkeratosis (thickening) of the periwound skin
- Subcutaneous hematoma with underlying full-thickness wound upon unroofing
- Poor quality of granulation tissue
- Variable drainage due to dependent position and/or presence of infection
- Presence of necrotic tissue, depending upon the vascular status

- Trophic skin changes (hair loss, thickened nails, pigment changes)
- Increased capillary refill time (>2 seconds is abnormal)
- Decreased response to direct pressure with monofilament testing
- Decreased or lack of pain[2]

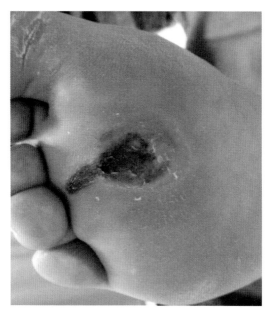

FIGURE 5-4. Following debridement, there is full-thickness ulceration on the plantar 3rd metatarsal head, which extends to the subcutaneous level (UT1A).

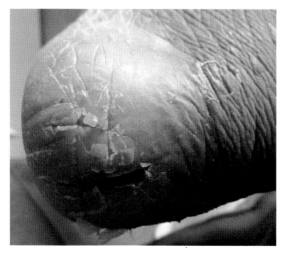

FIGURE 5-5. Fissure on the heel (UT1A).

Diagnostic Clue: Practitioners should be particularly sensitive to neuropathic patients with DFUs who report increased pain as this could be the hallmark of infection.

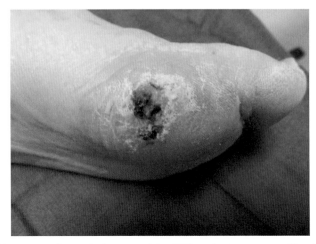

FIGURE 5-6. Hyperkeratotic tissue overlying DFU on the 1st metatarsal head (UT1A).

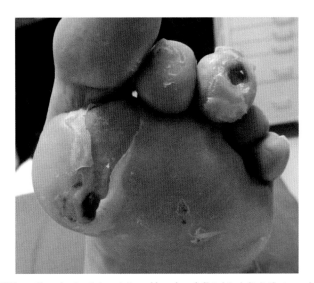

FIGURE 5-7. DFUs on the plantar 1st metatarsal head and distal 3rd digit that would need to be probed to determine depth of tissue involvement. Further testing may also be indicated to rule out infection.

Medical management
- Provide education and medical care tailored to the individual needs of the patient
- Refer to a vascular specialist for management of PAD[5]
- Refer to a podiatrist or foot/ankle specialist for surgical evaluation of foot deformities[6,7,8,9]
- Treat any infection present with both systemic antibiotics and topical agents[10]
- Confirm suspicious osteomyelitis with a bone biopsy.
- Refer to physical therapy for exercise (range of motion, strength, balance, and gait training)[11,12,13]
- Refer to a certified diabetic educator for education on diet and daily foot care, including foot inspection[14]

- After wound healing, refer to a pedorthotist for custom-fitted shoes to accommodate for residual bony abnormalities in order to prevent recurrence
- Replace dense foam inserts in any footwear every 3–6 months as they tend to "bottom out" and are no longer effective in pressure redistribution

> **Diagnostic Clue:** Erythema that extends >2 cm from the edge of a DFU is an indication that infection, not just critical colonization, may be present. Exposed bone in the wound bed (considered a positive probe-to-bone test) or a wound more than 2 cm² on the foot of a patient with diabetes, is suspicious of osteomyelitis and needs to be confirmed with further testing.

Wound management
- Debride the wound of all necrotic tissue and surrounding hyperkeratotic skin[15]
- Apply a dressing that will manage exudate and provide a topical antimicrobial agent[8,16]

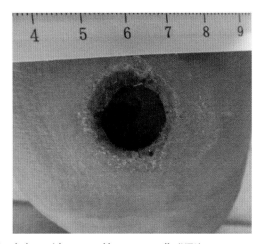

FIGURE 5-8. Deep heel ulcer with exposed bone, centrally (UT2).

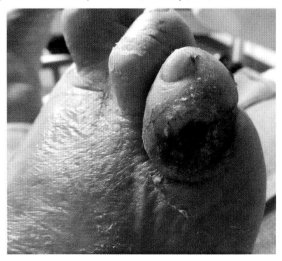

FIGURE 5-9. DFU that needs debridement and probing to determine tissue depth (UT2).

- Apply an appropriate off-loading device; non-removable devices such as the total contact cast (TCC) or irremovable cast walkers which have been shown to have the best results.[17,18,19] TCC application on patients with PAD is safe if the ankle pressure is ≥ 80 mm Hg, toe pressure is ≥ 74 mm Hg, ankle-brachial index is ≥ 0.55, or toe-brachial index is ≥ 0.55.[20] TCC is contraindicated in the presence of wound infection until the infection is treated effectively.
- Consider use of biologic skin substitutes as an adjunct to standard care when the wound is clean and granulating[21,22]

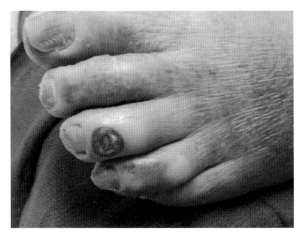

FIGURE 5-10. DFU on dorsal 3rd digit with signs of capsule involvement and infection (erythema, "sausage" toe, exposed necrotic bone) (UT2B).

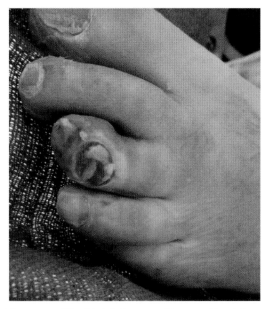

FIGURE 5-11. DFU with osteomyelitis of 3rd digit, exposed bone, and local signs of infection (UT3B).

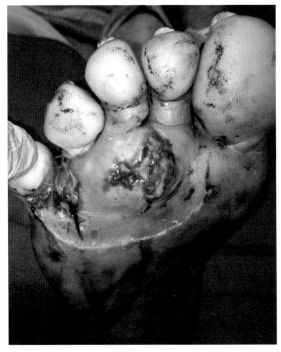

FIGURE 5-12. Deep plantar forefoot ulcer with tendon involvement and localized infection (UT2B).

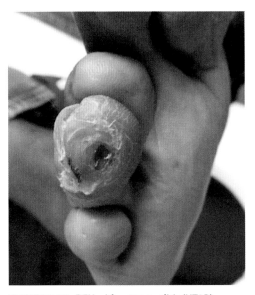

FIGURE 5-13. DFU with osteomyelitis (UT3B).

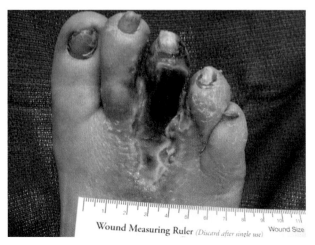

FIGURE 5-14. Deep interdigital wound with exposed tendon and ischemia (UT2C).

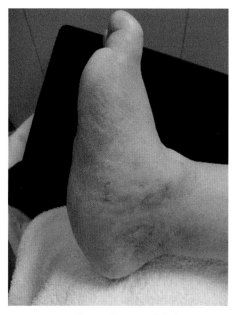

FIGURE 5-15. Charcot foot, medial view.

Clinical Guideline: Standard care requires definitive care of the DFU within 4 weeks of onset in order to prevent further tissue breakdown, infection, and progression to amputation. Wounds that do not reduce in size by 50% in the first 4 weeks of treatment are unlikely to heal in a reasonable period of time and adjunct therapies are recommended.[2,23]

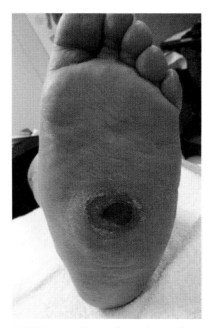

FIGURE 5-16. Charcot foot, plantar view.

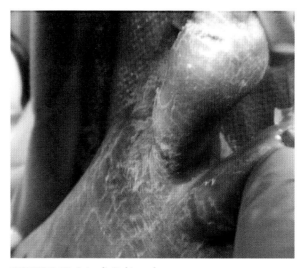

FIGURE 5-17. Interdigital toe ulcer.

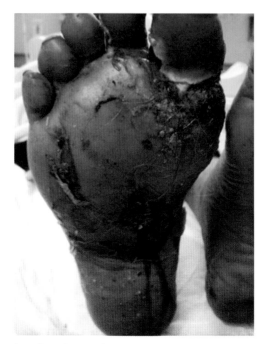

FIGURE 5-18. DFU with probe to bone/infection/ischemia (UT3D).

DIABETIC DERMOPATHY (ALSO TERMED PIGMENTED PRETIBIAL MACULES)

Figure 5-19

Pathophysiology
- Microvascular disease with reduced blood flow to the skin[24]
- May be related to mechanical or thermal trauma[25]
- Histologic changes of fibroblastic proliferation, thickening of collagen bundles, and fragmentation or separation of the collagen fibers[26]

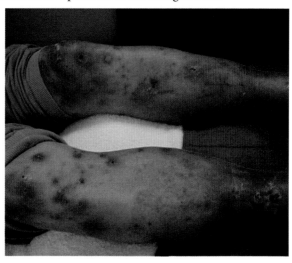

FIGURE 5-19. Diabetic dermopathy.

Clinical presentation
- Atrophic, hyperpigmented, well-demarcated macules on the skin[22]
- Healed ulcers with hypopigmented centers[22]
- May have erythema and scales[22]
- Bilateral asymmetrical distribution[22]
- Typically located on the shins[27]
- Lower extremity edema[22]

Medical management
- Tight control of blood sugars[28]
- Frequent dermatologic and musculoskeletal examinations[29]

Wound management
- Educate patients that wounds will heal spontaneously; however, new ones may form
- Provide education and resources on good skin care to prevent infection of open areas

ACKNOWLEDGEMENT

Reviewed by Adam L. Isaac, DPM & David G. Armstrong, DPM, MD, PhD.

REFERENCES

1. Davies MJ, D'Allessio DA, Fradkin J, Kernan WN, Mathieu C, Mingrone G, et al. Management of hyperglycemia in Type 2 diabetes, 2018: A concensus report by the American Diabetes Association (ADA) and the European Association for the Study of Diabetes (EASD). *Diabetes Care.* Available at https://care.diabetesjournals.org/content/41/12/2669. Accessed December 23, 2019.
2. Scarborough P, McGuire J. Diabetes and the diabetic foot. In Hamm R, ed. *Text and Atlas of Wound Diagnosis and Treatment.* 2nd ed. New York: McGraw Hill Education. 2019;199-233.
3. Armstrong DG, Lavery LA, Harkless LB. Validation of a diabetic wound classification system: the contribution of depth, infection, and ischemia to risk of amputation. Diabetes Care. 1998;21(5):855-859.
4. Mills Sr JL, Conte MS, Armstrong DG, Pomposelli FB, Schanzer A, Sidawy AN, ... & Society for Vascular Surgery Lower Extremity Guidelines Committee. The society for vascular surgery lower extremity threatened limb classification system: risk stratification based on wound, ischemia, and foot infection (WIfI). J Vasc Sur. 2014;59(1):220-234
5. Hinchliffe RJ, Brownrigg JR, Andros G, Apelqvist J, Boydo EJ, Fitridge R, et al. Effectiveness of revascularization of the ulcerated foot in patients with diabetes and peripheral artery disease: a systematic review. *Diabetes Metab Res Rev.* 2016;32(Suppl 1):136-144.
6. Bonanno DR, Gilles EJ. Flexor tenotomy improves healing and prevention of diabetes-related toe ulcers: A systematic review. *J Foot Ankle Surg.* 2017;56(3):600-604.
7. Shazadeh SP, Jupiter DC, Phancbhavi V. A systematic review of current surgical interventions for Charcot neuroarthropathy of the midfoot. *J Foot Ankle Surg.* 2017;56(6):1249-1252.
8. Hingorani A, LaMuraglia GM, Henke P, Meissner MH, Loretz L, Zinszer KM, et al. The management of the diabetic foot: A clinical practice guideline by the Society for Vascular Surgeons in collaboration with the American Podiatric Medical Association and the Society of Vascular Medicine. *J Vasc Surg.* 2016;63(2):3S-21S.
9. Crowe CS, Cho DY, Kneib CJ, Morrison SD, Friedrich JB, Keys KA. Strategies for reconstruction of the plantar surface of the foot: A systematic review of the literature. *Plast Reconstr Surg.* 2019;143(3):1223-1244.

10. Tchero J, Kangambega P, Noubou L, Becsangele B, Fluieraru S, Teot L. Antibiotic therapy of diabetic foot infections: A systematic review of randomized controlled trials. *Wound Repair Regen.* 2018;26(5):381-391.

11. Searle A, Spink MJ, Ho A, Chuter VH. Association between ankle equinus and plantar pressures in people with diabetes. A systematic review and meta-analysis. *Clin Biomech (Bristol, Avon).* 2017;43(3):8-14.

12. Liao F, An R, Pu F, Burns S, Shen S, Jan YK. Effect of exercise on risk factors of diabetic foot ulcers: a systematic review and meta-analysis. *Am J Phys Med Rehabil.* 2019;98(2):103-116.

13. Matos M, Mendes R, Silva AB, Sousa N. Phsyical activity and exercise on diabetic foot related outcomes: a systematic review. *Diabetes Res Clin Pract.* 2018;139(5):81-90.

14. Van Netten JJ, Price PE, Lavery LA, Monteiro-Soares M, Rasmussen A, Jubiz Y, et al. Prevention of foot ulcers in the at-risk patient with diabetes: A systematic review. *Diabetes Metab Res Rev.* 2016;32(Suppl 1):84-98.

15. Elraiyah T, Domecq JP, Prutsky G, Tsapas A, Nabhan M, Frykberg RG, et al. A systematic review and meta-analysis of debridement methods for chronic diabetic foot ulcers. *J Vasc Surg.* 2016;63(Suppl 2):37S-45S.

16. Dumville JC, Lipsky BA, Hoey C, Cruciani M, Fiscon M, Xia J. Topical antimicrobial agents for treating foot ulcers in people with diabetes. *Cochrane Database Syst Rev.* 2017;14(6):CD011038.

17. Bus SA, van Deursen RW, Armstrong DG, Lewis JE, Caravaggi CF, Cavanagh PR, International Working Group on the Diabetic Foot. *Diabetes Metab Res Rev.* 2016;32 (Suppl 1):99-118.

18. De Oliveira AL, Moore Z. Treatment of the diabetic foot by offloading: A systematic review. *J Wound Care.* 2015;24(12):562-570.

19. Elraiyah, T, Domecq JP, Prutsky G, Tsapas A, Nabhan M, Frykberg RG, et al. A systematic review and meta-analysis of off-loading methods for diabetic foot ulcers. *J Vasc Surg.* 2016;63(Suppl 2):59S.e1-2.

20. Tickner A, Klinghard C, Arnold JF, Marmolejo V. Total contact cast use in patients with peripheral arterial disease: a case series and systematic review. *Wounds.* 2018;30(2):49-56.

21. Gordon AJ, Alfonso AR, Nicholson J, Chiu ES. Evidence for healing diabetic foot ulcers with biologic skin substitutes: A systematic review and meta-analysis. *Ann Plast Surg.* 2019;83(4S Suppl 1):S31-S44.

22. Santema TB, Poyck PP, Ubbink DT. Systematic review and meta-analysis of skin substitutes in the treatment of diabetic foot ulcers: Highlights of a Cochrane systematic review. *Wound Repair Regen.* 2016:24(4):737-744.

23. Snyder RJ, Cardinal M, Dauphinee DM, Stavosky J. A Post-hoc analysis of reduction in diabetic foot ulcer size at 4 weeks as a predictor of healing by 12 weeks. *Ostomy Wound Management.* 2010;56(3):44-50.

24. Brugler A, Thompson S, Turner S, Ngo B, Rendell M. Skin blood flow abnormalities in diabetic dermopathy. *J Am Acad Derm.* 2011;65(3):559-563.

25. Smith MA. Diabetic Dermopathy. In Usatine RP, Smith MA, Mayeaux, Jr. EJ, Chumley HS, eds. *The Color Atlas and Synopsis of Family Medicine.* 3rd ed. New York, NY: McGraw-Hill. http://accessmedicine.mhmedical.com/content.aspx?bookid=2547&sectionid=206782278. Accessed December 29, 2019.

26. George SMC, Walton S. Diabetic dermopathy. *Brit J Diabetes Vasc Dis.* 2014;14(3):95–97.

27. Morgan AJ, Schwartz RA. Diabetic dermopathy: A subtle sign with grave implications. *J Am Acad Derm.* 2008;58(3):447-451.

28. Afarwal S, Gaur N. Cutaneous manifestations of diabetes mellitus. *Indian Journal of Medical Specialties.* 2015;6(3):102-107.

29. Sjorazo AA. Nasiri M, Yazdanpanah L. Dermatolgical and musculoskeletal assessment f diabetic foot: A narrative review. *Diabetes & Metabolic Syndrome: Clinical Research & Reviews.* 2016;10(2):S158-S164.

6

Burns

INTRODUCTION

Dermal injury that is termed "burn" can occur from thermal (heat and cold), chemical, electrical, and radiation sources, and while the clinical presentations have some similarities, the medical management of each condition is unique and specialized. The transfer of kinetic energy from any of these sources to the cellular structures of the skin causes a local inflammatory state, and the extent of exposure to the offending source and the amount of tissue damage can also result in systemic pathophysiologic processes. There are two important factors common to all of these conditions. First, any damage to the skin disrupts the body's natural barrier from the external environment and its microbes; therefore, infection is of utmost concern in treating any burn wound. Second, there are individual patient factors that affect the ability to heal, including nutrition, oxygenation, fluid resuscitation, age, co-morbidities, and stress.[1] Each one of these factors has to be evaluated and treated in the overall management of patients with burn injuries. This chapter reviews the tissue and systemic changes that occur with each type of burn, the classification systems used to describe tissue damage, and the medical and wound management for each type of dermal destruction in order to preserve both function and esthetics for the patient.

Evaluation of a patient with a burn injury begins with determining the mechanism of burn, the anatomical location of tissue damage, and the total burn surface area (TBSA). Figures 6-1 and 6-2 illustrate the two methods used to determine TBSA—Rule of Nines and Lund and Browder chart. In addition, the Palmar Surface Area (PSA) technique equates the patient's own palm and fingers to 1% TBSA and is useful for smaller and scattered patterns.[2] The depth of penetration, TBSA, and location are used to determine those patients who need to be referred immediately to a regional burn center for a higher level of care[3] (Table 6-1). Burns that are >10% TBSA may require systemic treatment and resuscitation, beginning with ABC evaluation. Burns that involve more than 30% TBSA are more likely to develop a systemic inflammatory response syndrome (SIRS).[1] Tachycardia, labored breathing, or respiratory distress require immediate treatment with endotracheal intubation and mechanical ventilation.

Burns that include flame injury or explosions are suspicious for inhalation injury, especially those that occur in a burning structure or an enclosed space. Signs that are indicative of inhalation injury include facial burns, singed facial hair, coughing, hoarseness, voice changes, and stridor. A bronchoscopy may be indicated to confirm inhalation injury, carbon debris, or ulceration.

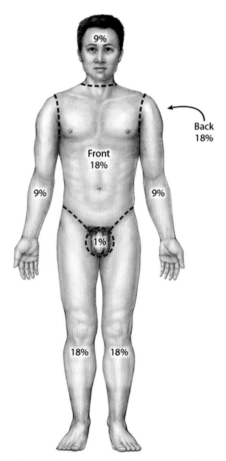

FIGURE 6-1. Rule of Nines. The Rule of Nines is used to determine total body surface area that is burned and estimates that each upper extremity accounts for 9 percent of the total burn surface area or TBSA, and each lower extremity, 18 percent. In addition, the anterior and posterior trunk is predicted to be 18 percent, the head and neck 18 percent, and the perineum 1%. For burns spanning anatomical regions, the volar surface area of the hand may be considered 1% of the TBSA.

Reproduced with permission from Hamm RL: *Text and Atlas of Wound Diagnosis and Treatment,* 2nd ed. New York, NY: McGraw Hill; 2019.

THERMAL BURNS

Pathophysiology
- Sources of heat include flames, scalding liquids, steam, and direct contact with a hot surface (e.g. iron or stove burner).
- Temperature of the heat source versus contact time is important in determining the amount of tissue injury, e.g. low temperatures for a long time or high temperature for a short time may cause a burn.
- Viscosity of the fluid affects the extent of tissue damage. Thicker fluids such as grease remain on the skin longer and can thereby cause more severe injuries. Water has a higher heat capacitance, stores more thermal energy, and can therefore cause greater damage per second of exposure. A combination of water and

oil causes the most damage because the oil prevents the water from evaporating.

- Areas covered by clothing will have more extensive injuries because the cloth absorbs the heated liquid, prevents heat dissipation by evaporation, and maintains contact with the skin for a longer period of time.
- Tar becomes adherent as it cools on the skin and creates a secondary alkaline chemical injury that requires special treatment, including removal of the tar with a solvent in order to prevent further tissue damage that will occur by pulling the tar off the skin.[4]
- The extent of a burn injury goes beyond the borders secondary to local inflammatory processes and is described in Figure 6-3.

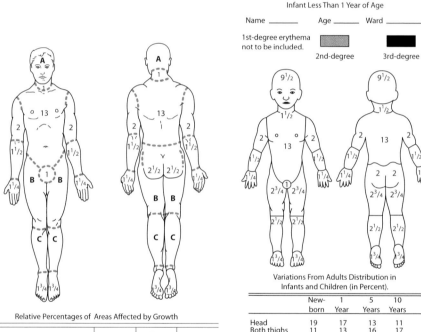

FIGURE 6-2. Lund and Browder chart. The Lund and Browder Chart is a more accurate method of determining the TBSA, and has separate scales for adults and children.

Reproduced with permission from Hay WW, Levin MJ, Absug MJ, et al: Current Diagnosis & Treatment: Pediatrics, 25th ed. New York, NY: McGraw Hill; 2020.

The table under the illustration is compiled from Berkow data.

TABLE 6-1.   American burn association criteria for referral to a regional burn center

- Partial-thickness or full-thickness burns that encompass > 10% TBSA in patients younger than 10 years or older than 50 years
- Partial-thickness or full-thickness burns > 20% TBSA in persons of other age groups
- Full-thickness burns > 5% TBSA in persons of any age group
- Burns that involve the face, hands, feet, genitalia, perineum, or major joints
- Electrical burns, including lightening injury
- Chemical burns
- Inhalation injury
- Burn injury in patients with pre-existing conditions that can complicate management, prolong recovery, or affect mortality
- Any patients with burns and concomitant trauma, in which burn injury poses the greatest risk of morbidity and mortality. If the trauma poses the greater immediate risk, the patient may be treated in a trauma center until stable, and then transferred to a burn center.
- Burn children in hospitals without qualified personnel or equipment for pediatric care
- Burn injury in patients who require special social, emotional, or rehabilitative intervention, including cases involving suspected child abuse or substance abuse

Data from www.ameriburn.org; Sheridan RL, Geibel J. What are the American Burn Association burn center transfer criteria? Chicago, IL: American Burn Association.

Clinical Guideline: Any child that presents with an immersion scald injury with symmetrical distribution on bilateral extremities and/or crease-sparing of the perineum and buttocks warrants suspicion of abuse and should be reported to a child protective agency.[2]

Clinical presentation
The American Burn Association has classified burns according to depth of tissue injury; following are the clinical characteristics of each classification.
- Superficial
  Figure 6-4
  o Involves only the epidermis without disruption of epithelial integrity
  o Presents with blanching erythema secondary to local capillary vasodilation
  o Heals in 3–4 days with desquamation of the damaged epithelium which is replaced by regenerating keratinocytes
- Superficial partial thickness
  Figures 6-5 and 6-6
  o Extends into the papillary dermis
  o Blanches with pressure
  o Typically forms a serum-filled blister as a result of the inflammatory process between the epidermis and dermis
  o May deepen after a few days, termed conversion or secondary deepening

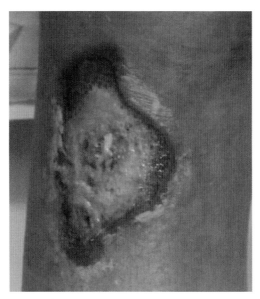

FIGURE 6-3. **Jackson's zones of injury.** Jackson's burn theory classifies three concentric zones of tissue viability. The zone of coagulation in the center is the area of maximum contact to the heat source. Tissue in this area undergoes a coagulation necrosis as proteins of the extracellular matrix are denatures and vascularity is impaired. Cells in this area will not recover and early debridement is an integral part of treatment in order to facilitate healing and to prevent infection. The zone of stasis is characterized by hypoperfusion and hypometabolism as the number of viable cells is substantially reduced. The area presents with blanching erythema and there is a risk of progression to necrosis if tissue perfusion is not preserved by the following treatment strategies: fluid resuscitation, avoidance of vasoconstrictors, and prevention of infection. Patients with comorbidities that impair blood flow (e.g. diabetes, PAD, tobacco use) are at increased risk for irreversible tissue damage. The outer zone of hyperemia, erythema as a result of local vasodilation, is completely viable and will recover if protected from further trauma and/or infection.

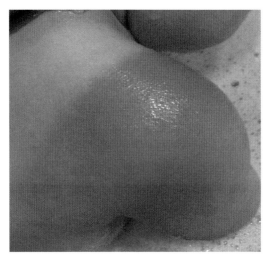

FIGURE 6-4. Superficial burn caused by sun overexposure.

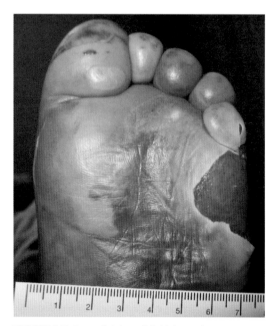

FIGURE 6-5. Superficial partial thickness burn.

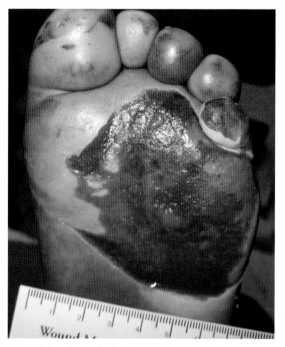

FIGURE 6-6. Superficial partial thickness burn reepithelializing.

- ◦ Remains sensate to pain, proprioception, and light touch
- ◦ Heals within 2–3 weeks by re-epithelialization from intact dermal appendages
- ◦ Rarely forms hypertrophic scars and/or wound contractures
- ◦ Does not require excision and grafting[2]

- Deep partial thickness
  Figures 6-7 and 6-8
  - ◦ Extends into the reticular dermis
  - ◦ Is nociceptively insensate

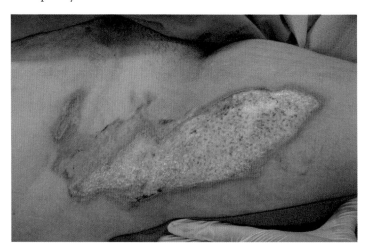

FIGURE 6-7. Deep partial thickness burn.

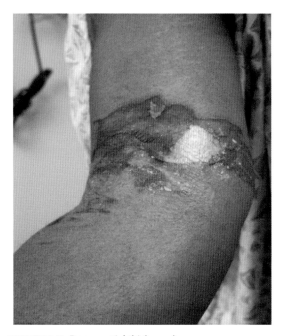

FIGURE 6-8. Deep partial thickness burn.

- o Has mottled white appearance or is pink
- o Does not blanche with pressure
- o May remain sensate to light touch, vibration and rapid pressure, stretch and sustained pressure (these receptors are deeper in the dermis and may be spared)
- o Heals in 3–9 weeks because of damage to the stem cell-containing hair follicles and sebaceous glands, as well as reticular fibroblasts
- o Healing by contracture will cause hypertrophic scarring and contractures with cosmetic and functional impairments
- • Full thickness

  Figure 6-9
  - o Extends through the dermis and across the subdermal plexus with complete loss of the skin's barrier function
  - o Obliterates all dermal regenerative cells
  - o Does not heal from the wound base
  - o Appears as white (due to scalding), leathery brown, or black eschar (due to flames) with no capillary refill[4]
  - o Has fixed pigmentation with no blanching
  - o Shrinks or contracts because the burn tissue is nonviable
  - o Is insensate to all forms of somato-sensation
  - o Has three concentric zones of tissue loss as defined by Jackson's burn theory (Figure 6-3)

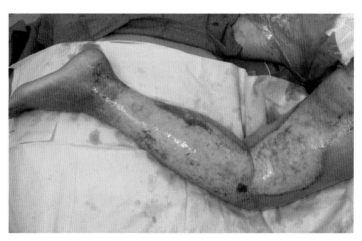

FIGURE 6-9. Full thickness burn.

Diagnostic Clue: When assessing a burn for depth, a helpful guide is "dead tissue shrinks, damaged tissue swells." Thus shrinking dead tissue would be classified as full thickness, and edematous burned tissue would be classified as partial thickness, either superficial or deep.

Medical management
- Superficial
  - Do not include in TBSA.
  - Hydrate if burn is extensive and patient complains of systemic symptoms (e.g. chills, headache).
  - Advise pain relievers as needed.

- Superficial partial thickness
  - Drain blisters and debride the skin in order to determine the depth.
  - Apply topical antimicrobial dressings.
  - Avoid prophylactic systemic antibiotics to prevent predisposition to colonization of multi-drug resistant organisms.[2]

- Deep partial thickness (burns that do not re-epithelialize in 2 weeks)
  - Remove rings and other jewelry or clothing that may act as a tourniquet.
  - Do not apply silver sulfadiazine prior to referral to burn center; it will have to be removed for assessment and may change the visual aspect of the wound by creating a "pseudo-eschar" covering.[4]
  - Debride necrotic tissue by direct excision or by enzymatic debridement.
  - Close with autologous skin grafting after surgical excision.
  - Refer to physical therapy for any burns that impair function.

- Full thickness
  - Assess for airway stability using the ABCs of trauma evaluation.
  - Triage to critical care and/or a burn center using the guidelines in Table 6-1.
  - Examine diaphragmatic dynamics and chest wall mechanics during respiration if there is circumferential or full-thickness injury to the torso, in which case an escharotomy may be indicated.[2]
  - Examine pulses frequently in any extremity with a circumferential burn; any decrease in pulses or neuromuscular integrity warrants immediate escharotomy.
  - Initiate fluid resuscitation for any patient with full-thickness burns over more than 20% TBSA.
  - Assess nutritional requirements for any patient with burns more than 30% TBSA in adults and 20% TBSA in children.[2]
  - Provide adequate pain medications sufficient to manage pain, yet allow patient to participate in dressing changes and rehabilitation tasks.
  - Initiate rehabilitation services as soon as patient is medically stable.

Wound management
- Superficial
  - Run cool tap water (between 2°C and 15°C) over the burn area; do not use ice.[1]
  - Apply a water-soluble cream containing aloe vera as needed to keep skin moist and to help alleviate pain.
  - Avoid sun exposure, tight clothing, or jewelry that will further damage the skin.

- Superficial partial thickness
  - Remove any non-viable debris.
  - Apply moist antimicrobial dressings sufficient to absorb any drainage.
  - Change dressings as needed to prevent periwound maceration.
  - Instruct in range of motion exercises for any burns that involve a joint.

- Deep partial thickness
  - Apply moist antimicrobial dressings after debridement; if using a silver dressing, soak in sterile water, not normal saline, because the chlorine ions will attach to silver ions and reduce the amount of silver delivered to the wound bed.[1]
  - Use a dressing that will accommodate the drainage and prevent maceration of the periwound skin, especially in the zone of hyperemia.
  - Use antimicrobial dressings for at least 48 hours post injury, then discontinue antimicrobial agent if there are no signs of infection.[1]
  - Avoid wet to dry dressings with gauze which can impair wound healing and destroy healthy cells upon removal!

- Full thickness
  - Apply moist antimicrobial dressings
  - Perform maintenance debridement as needed
  - Co-ordinate wound care with physician in order to prepare for grafting as soon as possible in order to minimize risk of infection and hypertrophic scarring

ELECTRICAL BURNS

Pathophysiology
The extent of the electric burn is related to the voltage, magnitude, frequency, type of current (alternating versus direct) and duration of the current flow, as well as the volume and resistance of the tissue through which the current passes.[2]

- Types of electrical burns
  - *Arc* occurs when the current passes from a high-resistance area to a low-resistance area; the electricity ionizes the air particles to complete the circuit so no contact with the skin is required to cause tissue damage. The heat generated is hot enough to ignite clothing, and the high-current arc can produce a pressure wave sufficient to throw an individual off balance and thereby cause injuries.
  - *Flash* occurs when an electrical arc (usually AC significantly higher than 50–60 Hz) passes over the skin, causing intense heat and light. Burns are mostly superficial over a large area with little or no damage to the subcutaneous tissue.
  - *Low voltage* occurs with <1000 V causing damage only to the tissues immediately surrounding the point of initial contact. Most low-voltage electrical burns involve either the hands or oral cavity from contact with an electrical cord that has no insulation.[5] Severity of the damage depends on the contact time.[2]
  - *High voltage* occurs with ≥1000 V; creates significant tetany that may result in bone fractures and myocyte necrosis which in turn leads to myoglobinuria, renal failure, and hyperkalemia, as well as possible life-threatening arrhythmias. Alternating current of 15–150 Hz may lead to tetanic contractions of the muscle that cause the "no-let-go" phenomenon, thereby causing more extensive subcutaneous injuries.[5]
  - *Flame* injury is caused by contact with objects that were ignited by an electrical source. Usually only involves the skin, not the deeper tissues.
  - *Oral* injury usually occurs only in children; caused by biting or chewing on an electrical cord. The current may travel from one side of the mouth to the other and thereby possibly cause a deformity.[6]
- Paths of resistance: current travels through tissues of least resistance [blood vessels, nerves, muscle, skin (wet < dry), tendon, fat, bone]. Because bone has

the most resistance, it accrues the most heat, thereby causing burn damage to the tissues (muscle, fascia, ligaments) surrounding the bone.

- Zones of electrical burns: occur around bone that absorbs enough heat to cause adjacent tissue damage; zones correspond roughly to Jackson's zones of cutaneous burns
  - Zone of necrosis—area of non-viable tissue adjacent to the heat source
  - Zone of ischemia—damaged tissue that is reversible if edema is managed
  - Zone of stasis—outer area that is viable if blood flow is maintained

The amount of tissue damage depends upon the magnitude and frequency of the current, length of exposure time, volume of tissue exposed (e.g. hands and feet have less soft tissue to dissipate the heat, so damage to these areas may be worse), and resistance of the tissue exposed to the current. Alternating current tends to cause more damage than direct current.[5]

Clinical presentation
- High-voltage entry wounds—charred, centrally depressed, leathery eschar
- High-voltage exit wounds—more "explosive" as the charge exits with more superficial tissue damage; may leave a black metallic coating on the skin that looks like eschar, due to vaporization of the metal contacts and electroplating of the conductive skin surface[3,5]
- Complaints of progressive pain on passive extension and/or paresthesia, indicative of compartment syndrome due to deep tissue damage around the bone
- Low-voltage hand burn—affects small area of the hand, usually in the line of contact with the wire (Figure 6-10)
- Lightning burns—cause direct current injury due to high heat (as much as 50,000° F) for a short period of time (1–2 milliseconds)
  - Lichtenberg figures—lacy ferning pattern on the superficial skin as a result of the flow of electrons over the body (Figure 6-11)
  - Punctate burns at the point of contact (Figure 6-12)
  - Most severe effect can be cardiac arrest and apnea[2]

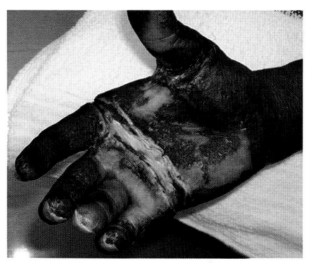

FIGURE 6-10. Electrical burn of the hand.
Reproduced with permission from Hamm RL: Text and Atlas of Wound Diagnosis and Treatment, 2nd ed. New York, NY: McGraw Hill; 2019.

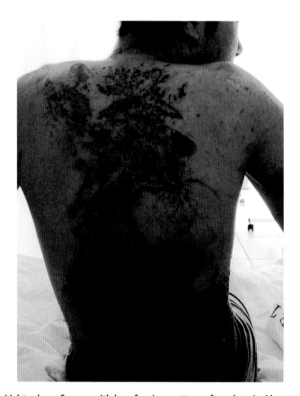

FIGURE 6-11. Lichtenberg figures with lacy ferning pattern after electrical burn on the upper chest.
Reproduced with permission from Ocak T, Duran A, Tekelioglu UY, et al: Two cases of lightning strikes resulting in Lichtenberg figures, 2014 March;32(1):37-38.

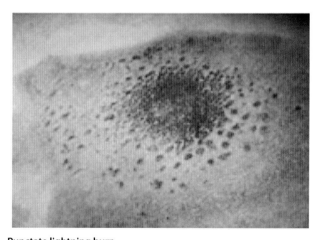

FIGURE 6-12. Punctate lightning burn.
Reproduced with permission from Knoop KJ, Stack LB, Storrow AB, et al: The Atlas of Emergency Medicine, 4th ed. New York, NY: McGraw Hill; 2016. Photo contributor: Arthur Kahn, MD.

Medical management
- Monitor for cardiac arrest, heart arrhythmias, and ventricular fibrillation for 48 hours post injury[2]
- Initiate aggressive fluid hydration.
- Correct any electrolyte imbalances.
- Initiate diuretics in order to minimize edema at the burn area.
- Monitor for signs of compartment syndrome and perform emergent fasciotomy if indicated.
- Evaluate for peripheral nerve injuries.
- Monitor sympathetic skin response for prediction of long-term bone loss. Amplitude threshold of 293.75 μV and latency of 2.15 sec has high sensitivity for predicting bone loss.[7]
- Transfer to a designated burn center when patient is stable.

Wound management
- Treat dermal injuries according to the guidelines under thermal burns. Assume that the total area of tissue damage may be much larger than the visible injury.
- Treat post-surgical fasciotomies with serial debridement, negative pressure wound therapy, or moist wound dressings (as recommended by plastic surgeon) until ready for surgical closure.

CHEMICAL BURNS

Figures 6-13 and 6-14

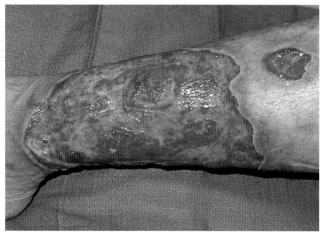

FIGURE 6-13. Venous wound being treated with acetic acid twice a day; the acid burns the healthy cells and inhibits wound healing.

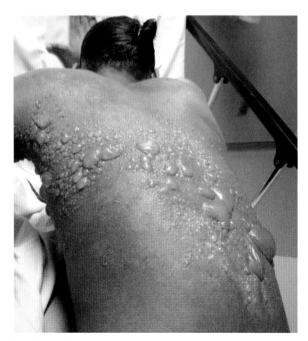

FIGURE 6-14. **Self-inflicted alkali burn with cleaner fluid.**
Reproduced with permission from Brunicardi FC, Andersen DK, Billiar TR, et al: Schwartz's Principles of Surgery, 11th ed. New York, NY: McGraw Hill; 2019.

Pathophysiology
- Caused by contact of the skin with strong acid or base solutions
- Occur most commonly on face, head, and hands
- Severity dependent upon the concentration of the agent, quantity and duration of contact, and other co-morbidities the victim may have
- Acidic burns—are less severe because contact results in coagulation necrosis of the tissue, thereby creating denatured protein eschar that impairs further penetration of the acid[2]
- Base or alkali burns—result in deeper injury because the agent causes liquefaction necrosis of the tissue, protein hydrolysis, and fat saponification, thereby creating a liquefied area of damage that allows the solution to penetrate underlying tissue[2]
- Hydrofluoric acid burns—cause liquefactive necrosis, deeper penetration of the acid solution, and therefore more tissue damage

Clinical presentation
- Redness, irritation, or burning at the site of contact
- Pain or numbness at the site of contact
- Blisters or black dead skin at the contact site
- Vision changes if the chemical gets into the eyes
- Cough or shortness of breath if the chemical is inhaled

Medical management
- Remove any contaminated clothing.
- Irrigate the affected area with copious amounts of water for at least 20 minutes with care not to let the water run over unaffected skin. Do not allow patient to sit in water.
- Call Poison Control at 1-800-222-1222 to determine if the chemical is toxic; refer to the chemical's material safety data sheet (MSDA) for recommended treatment protocols.
- Monitor for any systemic effects (shortness of breath, dizziness, nausea, and headache); treat appropriately.
- Manage any co-morbidities (diabetes, peripheral arterial disease, chronic venous insufficiency, etc.) to optimize wound healing.
- Provide adequate pain management.[8]

> **Clinical Guideline:** Diphoterine (a polyvalent, chelating, amphoteric hypertonic solution) has been shown to be safe and highly effective in improving healing time and pain management of chemical burns (both acidic and base) that occur on the skin and in the eyes, as compared with water or a physiologic solution equivalent, and is recommended to be readily available to emergency responders and in facilities where employees are exposed to hazardous chemical solutions.[9,10]

Wound management
- Remove any necrotic tissue
- Apply a moist wound dressing

FROSTBITE

Pathophysiology
- Caused by exposure to extremely low temperatures with resulting microvascular occlusion and subsequent tissue ischemia and cell death[11]
- Tissue damage occurs by the following interlinked processes:
  - Extracellular ice crystal formation as a direct injury
  - Resultant oncotic fluid shifts and intracellular dehydration
  - Vasoconstriction which causes microvascular thrombosis and tissue hypoxia
  - Reperfusion injury which increases endothelial damage
  - Cellular death and lysis with an increased inflammatory response[11,12]

Clinical presentation
- First degree, also called frostnip, affects only the epidermis and resolves with rewarming
  - White or red color of the affected skin
  - Numb feeling
  - May feel hard or stiff

- Second degree, also called superficial; affects the epidermis and dermis (Figure 6-15 and 6-16)
  - Initially red, then turns blue
  - Feels hard and frozen

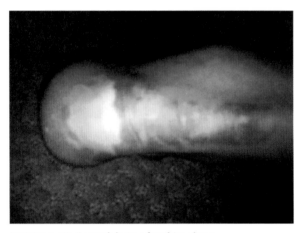

FIGURE 6-15. Second degree frostbite, day 1.

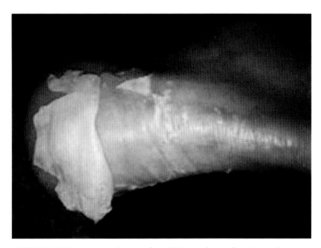

FIGURE 6-16. Second degree frostbite peeling after 1 week.

- ○ Forms blisters filled with clear or milky fluid
- ○ Edema of the affected area
- Third degree, also called deep, affects the epidermis, dermis, and subcutaneous tissue
  - ○ White, blue, or blotchy skin color
  - ○ Forms blisters that may be filled with blood
  - ○ Feels hard and cold
  - ○ Forms thick, black scabs over a period of weeks
- Fourth degree, also called deep, affects full-thickness skin, subcutaneous tissues, and deeper muscle, tendons, and bone (Figure 6-17)
  - ○ Initially deep red and mottled skin color that turns black
  - ○ Evidence of deeper tissue damage[13]
  - ○ Possible signs of compartment syndrome in the feet[14]

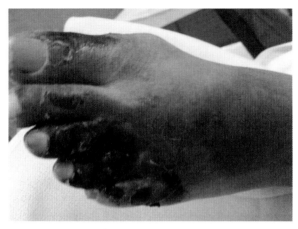

FIGURE 6-17. Deep frostbite.

Medical management
- Rapid rewarming with water immersion at 104°F to 108°F (40°C to 42°C) with care to avoid a thaw-freeze-thaw sequence that causes more tissue damage
- Tetanus prophylaxis
- Ibuprofen for anti-inflammatory effects
- Narcotic analgesics for pain control
- Tobacco and alcohol cessation[15]
- Monitoring for signs of compartment syndrome
- No debridement of necrotic tissue until edges of damaged tissue have completely demarcated[2]
- Intra-arterial thrombolysis with interventional radiology to evaluate perfusion[16], followed by systemic anticoagulation or antiplatelet therapy[17]
  - Recombinant tissue plasminogen activator (rt-PA) for fourth degree frostbite within 24 hours after rewarming
  - Iloprost within 48 hours after rewarming[18]
  - Prostacyclin for second to fourth degree frostbite within 48 hours of rewarming[19]
- Hyperbaric oxygen therapy to optimize tissue reperfusion after 24 hours[12]
- Triple phase bone scans to identify viable and non-viable bone in order to predict amputation sites, if indicated[20]

Wound management
- Aspiration and/or unroofing of blisters with clear or yellow fluid; no aspiration of hemorrhagic blisters
- Dry, sterile dressing (e.g. gauze pad or lamb's wool) between necrotic toes to prevent maceration
- Topical antimicrobial dressings on exposed wound beds after removal of any blisters[2,11]
- Standard moist wound care of any open wounds after debridement or amputation
- Referral to plastic surgeon for wound closure

RADIATION BURNS

Radiation therapy is an integral part of treating many malignant cancers because of its ability to destroy rapidly reproducing cells; however, there is a "by-stander" effect on the normal surrounding cells and tissues that manifests as dermal burns. The cancer cells receive radiation throughout the entire treatment time; the healthy cells receive the minimal amount possible. The resulting tissue damage is dependent on the type of energy source, total dose, time administered, and the location and size of the exposed field.[2] The radiation unit of absorbed radiation dose of ionizing radiation is termed the *gray*, defined as the absorption of one joule of ionizing radiation by one kilogram of matter, in this case human tissue. Skin damage can be immediate, acute, and delayed, and while immediate radiation burns are much like superficial burns (also termed acute radiation dermatitis), the acute and delayed damage is much more difficult to treat because the cells have lost their ability to repair tissue, and the effects of the radiation continue even after therapy has ceased. The effects of any given radiation treatment depend upon the following factors: dose, treatment volume, daily fraction size, energy and type of radiation, total treatment time, and individual cellular differences.[21]

Pathophysiology
- An electron is ejected from a targeted molecule resulting in the release of free radicals.
- The double-stranded DNA of the cell is broken, rendering the cell unable to replicate or repair.
- Radiation causes blood vessel dilation, increased capillary permeability, and activation of coagulation, resulting in necrosis of endothelial cells.
- An inflammatory response ensues with erythema and edema similar to a superficial burn and can progress to superficial and deep partial thickness injury.
- The immune behavior of the affected skin is compromised with destabilization of the immune control, leading to either reduced immunity or excess immunity. These areas are termed immunocompromised districts (ICD).[22]
- The irradiated skin areas have decreased or altered lymphatic flow with oncologic lymphedema.
- The ICD develops dysfunction of neuro-immune signaling due to fibrotic throttling or reduction of peptidergic nerve fibers, resulting in a significant dysregulation of the local immune system and increased risk of infections.[22]

Clinical presentation
- Immediate
  Figures 6-18 and 6-19
  - Initially appears as faint erythema
  - Becomes dry scaling skin, termed *dry desquamation,* which occurs with <30 grays of radiation
  - Resolves in 2–3 months with only slight pigmentation changes due to increased melanin in the skin

- Acute
  Figure 6-20 through 6-22
  - Occurs in third or fourth week of treatment
  - Appears as erythema localized to the radiation field with warmth and tenderness

- ○ Is edematous with small foci of hemorrhage due to arteriolar obstruction by the fibrin thrombi
- ○ May become *wet desquamation* with dose >40 grays, characterized by the following:
  - • Pain
  - • Bullae, edema, fibrinous exudate
  - • Reepithelialization after 10 days if there is no infection

- ○ May ulcerate with full-thickness skin loss, eschar, and non-viable subcutaneous tissue
- ○ Frequent recurrence of open wounds[23]

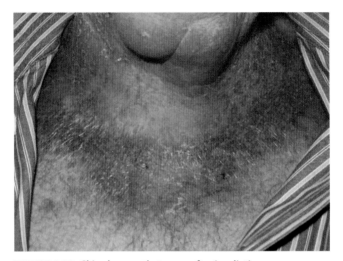

FIGURE 6-18. Skin changes that occur after irradiation.

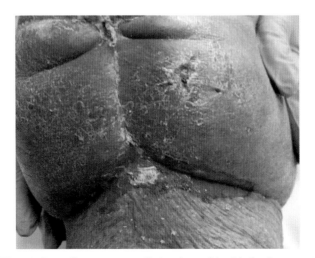

FIGURE 6-19. Immediate or acute radiation dermatitis with dry desquamation.

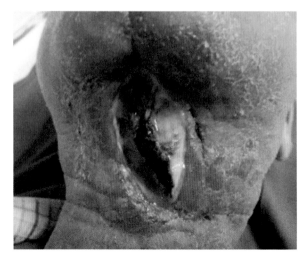

FIGURE 6-20. Acute open wound after radiation therapy to the neck.

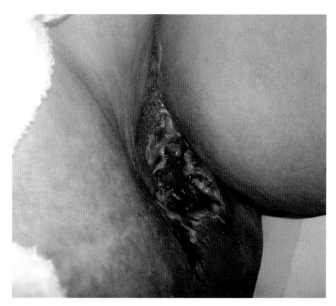

FIGURE 6-21. Full-thickness skin loss with eschar and surrounding erythema after radiation to the axillary region. Changes in skin color are visible distal to the open wound.

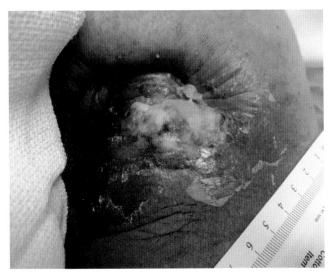

FIGURE 6-22. Full thickness skin loss and wet desquamation after radiation to the throat.

- Chronic
  Figures 6-23 and 6-24
  - Skin changes that include loss of hair, pigmentation changes, telangiectasia, and impaired vascularity
  - May develop osteoradionecrosis
  - May develop secondary malignancies
  - Impaired wound healing with trauma to the irradiated area; may occur months to years after radiation

Medical management
- Use of a thin silicone film dressing during radiation to help reduce incidence and severity of ARD[24]
- No surgical therapy indicated for acute wounds
- Surgical referral for osteoradionecrosis or chronic infection
- Surgical removal of all affected tissue and replacement with healthy tissue, usually including a flap transfer from an unaffected area with adequate blood supply and healthy epithelium
- Application of stem cell therapy for radiation-induced chronic wounds[25]
- Hair follicle transplants as a source of healthy stem cells for superficial, clean chronic wounds.

Wound management
- Application of topical corticosteroids to ARD may reduce symptoms of itching and reduce the likelihood of wet desquamation.[26]
- Apply an aloe-based cream to moisturize irradiated skin.
- Educate patient to avoid sun exposure, friction, shear, and other mechanical forces on irradiated tissue (e.g. by wearing loose clothing).
- Palliative care for extensive chronic wounds that cannot be surgically closed,

consisting of thin silicone-backed primary dressings and absorbent secondary dressings, anchored with silicone-backed or hypoallergenic tape, gauze rolls, or other non-adhesive material. (Figure 6-25)

- Biophysical modalities are contra-indicated in almost all cases of malignancy; however, negative pressure wound therapy may be used for palliative care in some cases.

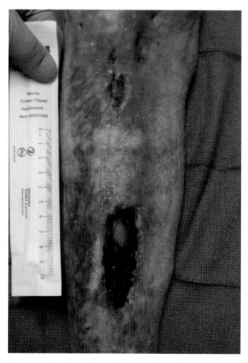

FIGURE 6-23. Chronic wound with osteoradionecrosis and permanent skin changes, occurs months to years after radiation therapy.

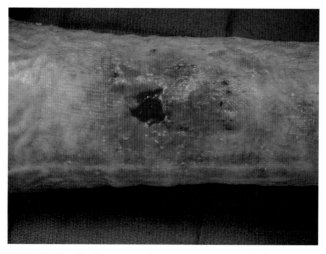

FIGURE 6-24. Non-healing traumatic wound on previously irradiated tissue.

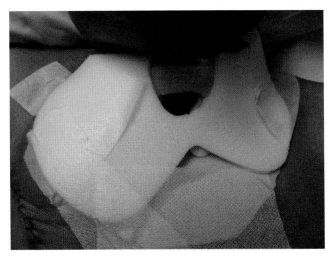

FIGURE 6-25. Use of silicone-backed foam dressings and hypoallergenic tape to manage drainage of an acute, nonhealing radiation wound.

REFERENCES

1. Khosroshahi AF, Had JS, Kheirjou R, Ranjkesh MR, Roshangar L. Skin burns: Review of molecular mechanisms and therapeutic approaches. *Wounds.* 2019;31(12):308-315.
2. Collier ZJ, Pham C, Carey JN, Gillenwater J. Burn Wound Management. In Hamm R, ed. *Text & Atlas of Wound Diagnosis and Treatment.* New York: McGraw Hill Education. 2019;299-319.
3. Sheridan RL, Geibel J. What are the American Burn Association burn center transfer criteria? *Medscape.* Available at https://www.medscape.com/answers/435402-117240/what-are-the-american-burn-association-burn-center-transfer-criteria. Posted 1/10/18. Accessed January 18, 2020.
4. Hermans MHE. An introduction to burn care. *Advances in Skin & Wound Care.* 2019;32(1):9-18.
5. Vande Ven H, Narayan D. Electrical Burn Injuries. Available at https://emedicine.medscape.com/article/1277496-overview#a2. Accessed January 31, 2020.
6. https://en.wikipedia.org/wiki/Electrical_burn. Accessed 1/31/20.
7. Roshanzamir S, Keshavarzi E. Sympathetic skin response impairment: a good predictor of bone loss in electrical burn victims. *Burns.* 2019. Available at doi: 10.1016/j.burns.2019.07.034. Accessed February 4, 2020.
8. Chemical burns. Available at https://www.webmd.com/first-aid/chemical-burns#3-8. Accessed February 4, 2020.
9. Lynn DD, Zukin LM, Dellavalle R. The safety and efficacy of Diphoterine for ocular and cutaneous burns in humans. *Cutan Ocul Toxicol.* 2017;36(2):185-192.
10. Alexander KS, Wasiak J, Cleland H. Chemical burns: Diphoterine untangled. *Burns.* 2018;44(4):752-766.
11. Ghumman A, Malic C. A novel application for Aquacel Ag in paediatric frostbite. *Burns Open.* Available at https://doi.org/10.1016/j.burnso.2018.06.002. Accessed February 6, 2020.
12. Ghumman A, St. Denis-Katz H, Ashton R, Wherrett C, Malic C. Treatment of frostbite with hyperbaric oxygen therapy: A single center's experience of 22 cases. *Wounds.* 2019;31(12):322-325.

13. Harding M. Frostbite. Available at https://patient.info/signs-symptoms/frostbite-leaflet. Accessed February 6, 2020.
14. Brandao R, St John JM, Langan TM, Schneekloth BJ, Burns PR. Acute compartment syndrome of the foot due to frostbite: Literature review and case report. *J Foot Ankle Surg.* 2018;57(2):382-387.
15. McCauley RL, Hing DN, Robson MC, Heggers JP. Frostbite injuries: A rational approach based on the pathophysiology. *J Trauma.* 1983;23(2):143-147.
16. Mullen M, Zachary T, Foley R, Irani Z. Thrombolysis for frostbite: A case study and clinical considerations. *Journal of Radiology Nursing.* 2019; 38(4):237-240.
17. Jones LM, Coffey RA, Natwa MP, Bailey JK. The use of intravenous tPA for the treatment of severe frostbite. *Burns.* 2017;43(5):1088-1096.
18. Pandey P, Vadlamudi R, Pradhan R, Pandey KR, Kumar A, Hackett P. Case report: severe frostbite in extreme altitude climbers – The Kathmandu iloprost experience. *Wilderness & Environmental Medicine.* 2018;29(3):366-374.
19. Cauchy E, Davis CB, Pasquier M, Meyer EF, Hackett PH. A new proposal for management of severe frostbite in the austere environment. *Wilderness & Environmental Medicine.* 2016;27(1):92-99.
20. Shenaq DS, Gottlieb LJ. Cold injuries. *Hand Clin.* 2017;33(2):257-267.
21. Gosselin TK, Schneider SM, Plambeck MA, Rowe K. A prospective randomized, placebo-controlled skin care study in women diagnosed with breast cancer undergoing radiation therapy. *Oncology Nursing Forum.* 2010;37(5):619-626.
22. Ruocco E, Di Maio R, Caccavale S, Siano M, Schiavo AL. Radiation dermatitis, burns, and recall phenomena: Meaningful instances of immunocompromised district. *Clinics in Dermatology.* 2014;32(5):660-669.
23. Mendelsohn FA, Divino CM, Kerstein ED. Wound care after radiation therapy. *Advances in Skin & Wound Care.* 2002;15:216-224.
24. Report of clinical trial. Available at https://clinicaltrials.gov/ct2/show/NCT03910595. Accessed February 29, 2020.
25. Rigotti G, Marchi A, Galie M, et al. Clinical treatment of radiotherapy tissue damage by lipoaspirate transplant: A healing process mediated by adipose-derived adult stem cells. *Plastic Reconstr Surg.* 2007;119(5):1409-1422.
26. Haruna F Lipsett A, Marignol L. Topical managementof acute radiation dermatitis in breast cancer patients: A systematic review and meta-analysis. *Anticancer Res.* 2017;37(10):5343-5353.

7

Immune-Mediated Tissue Injury

INTRODUCTION

The goal of the immune system is to protect the body from anything that is not a part of it, from germs to foreign bodies to harmful substances. The exquisite process of immunology begins in the skin with cells that phagocytose bacteria (macrophages, polymorphic neutrophilic lymphocytes), cells that release cytokines (endothelial cells, activated platelets, neutrophils, and T-lymphocytes), and dendritic cells that carry antigens from the injury site to the local lymph nodes where the adaptive immune system is activated.[1] If the immune system is over-activated, the body will attack itself and destroy healthy cells and tissues; if it is suppressed, the body becomes susceptible to microbes that are normally destroyed and therefore it develops infections more easily.[2] While a discussion of this miraculous process is beyond the scope of this chapter, it is important to recognize that both the up- and down-regulation of the immune system and its processes can result in dermal wounds, *or* they can impede the healing of existing wounds through a change in cellular activity or as a result of the medication used to treat the disorder. The purpose of this chapter is to assist the clinician in recognizing wounds that are mediated by immune disorders, as well as to stress the importance of understanding the effects of medications (e.g. corticosteroids, NSAIDs, anti-rejection medications, and other immune-suppressors) on the wound healing process, in which case collaboration between the wound care clinician and the immunologist is needed to manage the medications in such a way that wound healing is optimized.

HYPERSENSITIVITY SYNDROMES

An allergic reaction can be either contact (the offending substance comes in direct contact with the skin) or systemic (the offending substance is either injected or ingested). In either case, the offending substance is lysed or broken down by the macrophages and polymorphic neutrophilic lymphocytes (PMNs), and the resulting antigens (*anti*body *gen*erators) are presented to the host immune system T cells, thereby activating the complex immune response. Reactions can vary from mild to life-threatening, and will usually increase in severity with multiple exposures to the offending agent. The first treatment of any allergic reaction is to identify and stop use of the offending substance. Table 7-1 lists common agents for both allergic contact dermatitis and irritant contact dermatitis, and Table 7-2 lists medications that are most commonly reported to cause drug-induced hypersensitivity syndromes.

TABLE 7-1.   Common Allergens For Contact Dermatitis

Contact allergens
- Neomycin
- Bacitracin
- Wool
- Alcohol
- Formaldehyde
- Parabens
- Tape adhesives
- Latex
- Perfumes
- Metals (e.g. nickel, silver)

Irritant allergens
- Soap
- Detergent
- Cleaning solvents
- Poison ivy or oak
- Pesticides

Among both the adult and pediatric populations, the most common contact allergen is nickel.[3,4] In the adult population, nickel was followed by fragrance mix, cobalt, Myroxylon pereirae (Balsam of Peru, a natural mixture of resins and essential oils), chromium, p-phenylenediamine (PPD, a common ingredient in hair dyes), methylchloroisothiazolinone/methylisothiazolinone (MCI/MI, common chemicals in household items and skin care products), and colophonium (gum rosin used in hair removers).[3] In children, the most common contact allergens (after nickel) were ammonium persulfate (a potent oxidizing agent), gold sodium thioisulfate (used in gold jewelry), thimerosal (also known as Merthiolate, a preservative used in vaccines), and toluene-2,5-diamine (p-toluenediamine, a common cosmetic and hair dye ingredient).[4] As indicated, the offending substance is often embedded in common, everyday products and thus may be difficult to identify. Therefore, an in-depth, thorough subjective history is often required in order to identify the source of the allergic reaction.

CONTACT DERMATITIS

Figures 7-1 through 7-8

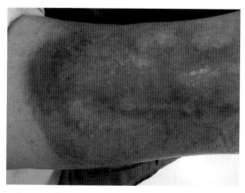

FIGURE 7-1. Contact dermatitis caused by elastic in a compression wrap.

TABLE 7-2. Most commonly reported medications that cause drug-induced hypersensitivity syndrome

Drug Class	Specific Drug	Latent Period
Angiotensin-converting enzyme inhibitors	Captopril	At any time
Xanthine oxidase inhibitor	Allopurinol	2–6 weeks
Antibiotics	Beta-lactams (pediatrics)	Immediate: 1 hour Non-immediate: ≥1 hour
	Ceftriaxone	72 hours
	Cyclosporine	
	Dapsone	Few days to weeks
	Isoniazid	
	Levofloxacin	
	Minocycline	
	Penicillin	
	Sulfonamides	
	Trimethoprim	
Anticonvulsants	Carbamazepine	Usually 2–4 weeks; may be to 3 months
	Lamotrigine	
	Phenobarbitone	
	Phenytoin	
	Primidone	
Antidepressants	Clomipramine (anafranil)	
Antifungals	Terbinafine	2–3 days
Antiretrovirals	Abacavir	
	Nevirapine	
Beta-blocker	Atenolol	
Biologic modifiers	Infliximab	
	Murine and humanized monoclonal antibodies	
	Recombinant interferons	
Drug coloring agents	Blue dyes	
Calcium channel blockers	Diltiazem	2–3 days
Gold salts		
Antihypertensive	Hydralazine (apresoline)	
Immunosuppressants	Azathioprine	
Non-steroidal anti-inflammatory drugs	Aspirin	
Antiarrhythmic	Procainamide	
Sodium channel blockers	Mexiletine	
Disease-modifying anti-rheumatic drugs	Sulfasalazine	

Reproduced with permission from Hamm RL: Drug allergy: delayed cutaneous hypersensitivity reactions to drugs, EMJ Allergy Immunol. 2016 Aug 2;1[1]:92-101.

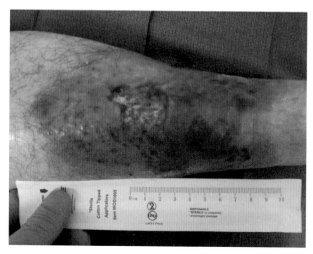

FIGURE 7-2. Contact dermatitis caused by a silver dressing.

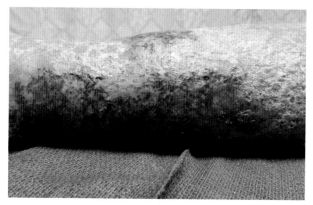

FIGURE 7-3. Contact dermatitis caused by a silicone-backed dressing under compression therapy.

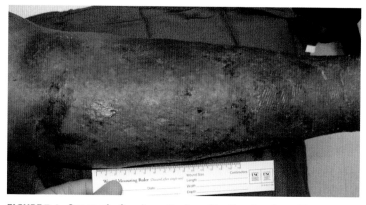

FIGURE 7-4. One week after discontinuing offending dressing with continued compression therapy.

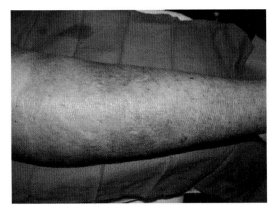

FIGURE 7-5. Complete healing with elimination of offending dressing with continued compression.

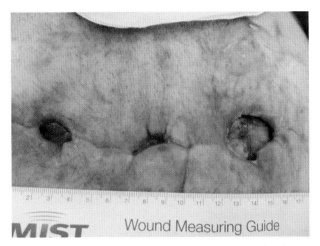

FIGURE 7-6. Contact allergic reaction to transparent film adhesive used with negative pressure therapy.

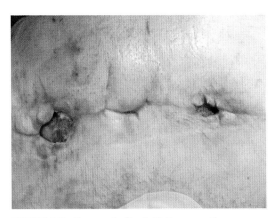

FIGURE 7-7. One week after initiating negative pressure wound therapy holiday.

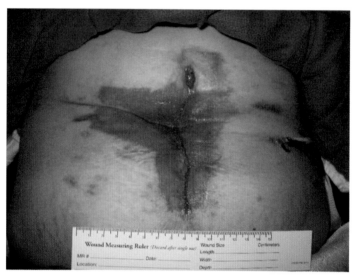

FIGURE 7-8. Allergic reaction (combination of contact and irritant) to both the adhesive used with negative pressure wound therapy and the caustic drainage from an enterocutaneous fistula.

Pathophysiology
- Allergic contact dermatitis
  - Is a Type IV delayed-type hypersensitivity reaction resulting from the activation of allergen-specific T cells[5]
  - Depends upon the chemical, the duration and nature of contact, and susceptibility of the exposed individual[6]
- Irritant contact dermatitis
  - Is not an immunologic response
  - Is a reaction to a caustic substance (e.g. chemical substance, cleaning solutions, acids)
  - Is an inflammatory cascade initiated by keratinocytes producing cytokines upon exposure to the substance[7]
  - Severity of reaction depends upon the concentration of the substance

Clinical presentation
- Skin changes noted only in areas of direct contact with the allergen
- Erythema, weeping, scaling of the periwound area
- Pruritis
- In severe cases, shiny skin and alopecia

Medical management
- Identification and removal of the offending material
- Potent or moderately potent steroids for allergic contact dermatitis[8]
- Antihistamines to decrease inflammation and discomfort[9]

Wound management
- Prevention of irritant contact dermatitis
  - Barrier creams containing dimethicone or perfluoropolyethers

- ○ Diethylenetriamine pentaacetic acid (chelator) for nickel, chrome, and copper dermatitis
- ○ Cotton glove liners to protect the hands
- ○ Softened fabrics on the skin[8]
- Treatment of irritant contact dermatitis
  - ○ Lipid-rich moisturizers[8]
- Treatment of allergic contact dermatitis
  - ○ Low-dose topical steroid creams
  - ○ Non-adherent hypoallergenic dressings for treatment of open wounds that exhibit signs of allergic reactions to routine dressings
  - ○ Latex-free gloves for treatment of any patient who has a history of allergies

DRUG-INDUCED HYPERSENSITIVITY SYNDROME (DIHS)

Figures 7-9 through 7-11

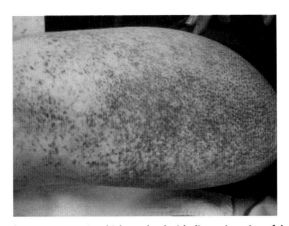

FIGURE 7-9. DIHS due to vancomycin which resolved with discontinuation of the medication.

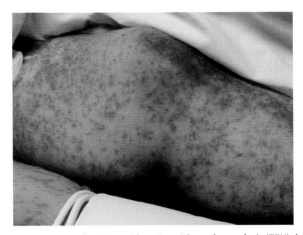

FIGURE 7-10. Lower extremity of patient with toxic epidermal necrolysis (TEN) due to an antibiotic.

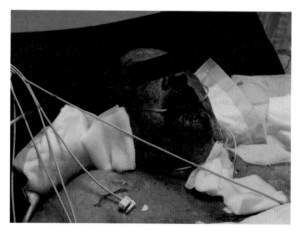

FIGURE 7-11. Upper body of patient with TEN.

Pathophysiology
- Is an immunologic response to a drug received either orally, by injection, or by IV (Table 7-2)
- Is similar to dermal allergic reactions except that the immune response is activated by the causative agents and their metabolites rather than by a direct effect on the keratinocytes
- Is a T cell-mediated hypersensitivity reaction that appears to be a result of impaired function of regulatory T cells which act to suppress the immune system (Tregs), and their effect on activation of drug-specific T effector cells[10]
- Involves specific polymorphisms in HLA genotypes that are drug specific
- Has various nomenclature based on symptoms (Table 7-3)

Clinical presentation
- Maculopapular rash that develops 3 weeks to 3 months after initiating a new drug
- Mucosal lesions and conjunctivitis (in more severe cases)
- Epidermal blistering and sloughing with a positive Nikolsky sign (in toxic epidermal necrolysis and Stevens-Johnson syndrome)
- Fever ($>38°$ C)
- Symptoms that continue after discontinuation of the causative drug
- Liver abnormalities (ALT >100 U/L)
- Presence of at least one of the following leukocyte abnormalities:
  - Leukocytosis ($>11 \times 10^9$/L)
  - Atypical lymphocytosis ($>5\%$)
  - Eosinophilia ($>1.5 \times 10^9$/L)
- Lymphademopathy
- HHV-6 reactivation (for DIHS in Asian population)[10]

TABLE 7-3. Nomenclature and symptoms for drug-induced hypersensitivity syndromes

Syndrome	Description
Erythema multiforme	Generalized rash with macular or papular skin eruptions; used to describe the syndrome in the younger adult population (20–40 years)
Drug rash with eosinophilia and systemic symptoms (DRESS)	Three of the following: fever, exanthema, eosinophilia, atypical circulating lymphocytes, lymphadenopathy, hepatitis
Stevens-Johnson syndrome	Cutaneous lesions of papules, vesicles, or bullae covering <10% of the body surface area; mucosal lesions; conjunctivitis
Toxic epidermal necrolysis	Cutaneous lesions of papules, vesicles, or bullae covering >30% of the body surface area; mucosal lesions; conjunctivitis
Acute generalized exanthematous pustulosis (AGEP)	Diffuse red or white pustules that appear 1–5 days after beginning a new medication; resolves within 1–3 days after stopping the offending medication
Chemotherapy-induced acral erythema	Painful swelling and erythema of the palms and soles of patients on high-dose chemotherapy
Drug-induced lupus erythematosus	Lupus-type symptoms with skin signs associated with medications; resolves when medications withdrawn.

Reproduced with permission from Hamm RL. Drug-hypersensitivity syndrome: diagnosis and treatment, J Am Coll Clin Wound Spec 2012 Jun 23;3(4):77-81.

Medical management
- Identification and cessation of the offending medication (usually the last one that the patient initiated taking)
- Systemic corticosteroids for the clinical symptoms, beginning with 40–50 mg/day and tapering over 6–8 weeks; continuation of corticosteroids for 2–3 months to prevent relapse[10]
- Treatment of any complications that occur (e.g. myocarditis, pneumonia, sepsis, gastrointestinal bleeding, renal dysfunction)
- Supportive care in an intensive care or burn unit for severe cases
- Pharmogenetic screening tests; e.g. HLA-B*5701 for abacavir[11], HLA-B*5801 for allopurinol[12], HLA-B*1301 for dapsone[13]

Wound management
- Wound management of epidermal sloughing similar to treatment of deep superficial burns
- Debridement of detached epidermal tissue generally not advised because of potential fluid loss
- Non-adherent antimicrobial dressings over open wounds
- Dressings to promote re-epithelialization as wounds progress

ATOPIC DERMATITIS

Figures 7-12 through 7-14

Pathophysiology
- Chronic, relapsing, non-contiguous, exudative eczema/dermatitis that affects 20–30% of all children and 7–10% of all adults[14,15]
- Impairment of the stratum corneum barrier resulting in altered skin function, an increase in trans-epidermal water loss, and dehydration[14]
- Inflammatory processes characterized by the production and release of several cytokines, chemokines, and interleukins with increased inflammation levels and risk of infections[14]
- Regarded as a T helper type 2 lymphocyte-mediated disease
- Likely progression to the "atopic march" of allergic rhinitis, asthma, and food allergies

Clinical presentation
- Chronic itching
- Dry skin with eczematous lesions
- Frequent recurrence of signs and symptoms

Medical management
- Topical creams (for patients over 2 years of age)
  - Corticosteroids
  - Calcineurin inhibitors (tacrolimus, pimecrolimus)[15]
- Oral antihistamines
- Short-term oral antibiotics if needed
- Oral corticosteroids for most severe cases
- Dupilumab (an injectable biologic)[15]
- Anti-IgE medication (omalizumab), for pediatric population per the ADAPT study[16]
- Some Janus kinase 1 inhibitors (e.g. upadacitinib) for adult moderate to severe cases[17]

Wound management
- Topical ointments to hydrate the skin, e.g. glycerol 85%[18]
- Narrow-band ultraviolet B therapy[19]
- Antimicrobial dressings for open wounds with exudate
- Infants
  - Avoid any skin irritants
  - Avoid extreme temperatures
  - Give warm baths followed by skin lubrication with lipid-based ointment[20,21]

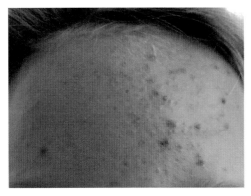

FIGURE 7-12. Atopic dermatitis on the forehead of a 10-year-old.

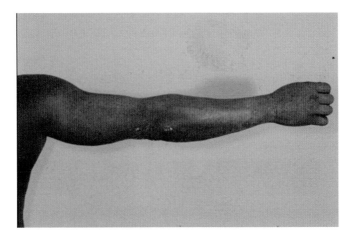

FIGURE 7-13. Atopic dermatitis on the upper extremity.

Reproduced with permission from Kelly AP, Taylor SC, Lom HW, et al: Taylor and Kelly's Dermatology for Skin of Color, 2nd ed. New York, NY: McGraw Hill; 2016.

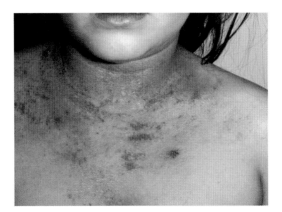

FIGURE 7-14. Atopic dermatitis on the upper chest of a child.

Reproduced with permission from Kelly AP, Taylor SC, Lom HW, et al: Taylor and Kelly's Dermatology for Skin of Color, 2nd ed. New York, NY: McGraw Hill; 2016.

VASCULITIS

Figures 7-15 through 7-23

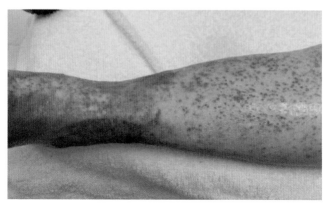

FIGURE 7-15. Vasculitis on the lower extremity.

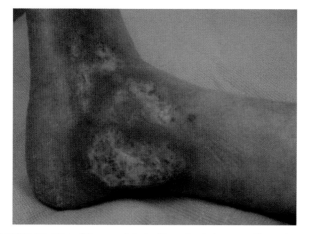

FIGURE 7-16. Vasculitis associated with systemic lupus erythematosus (SLE).

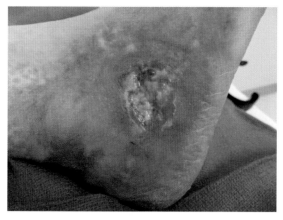

FIGURE 7-17. Vasculitis associated with SLE.

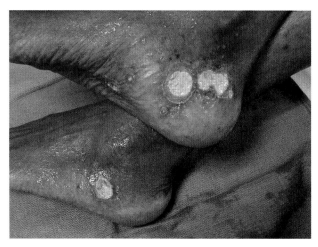

FIGURE 7-18. Vasculitis associated with SLE.

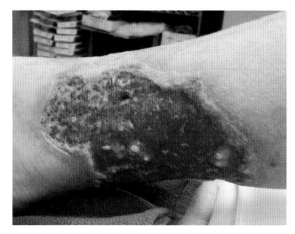

FIGURE 7-19. Vasculitis caused by polyarteritis nodosum.

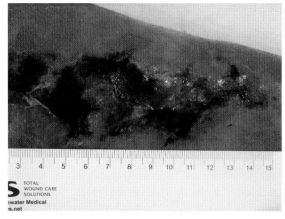

FIGURE 7-20. Vasculitis on lower extremity of a patient who had symptoms of cerebral involvement 2 weeks prior to skin necrosis.

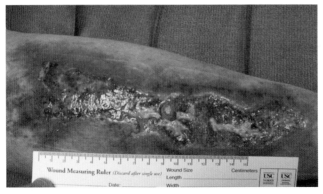

FIGURE 7-21. Vasculitis after 3 weeks of treatment with non-contact low-frequency ultrasound, non-adherent dressings, and compression therapy in addition to medical therapy.

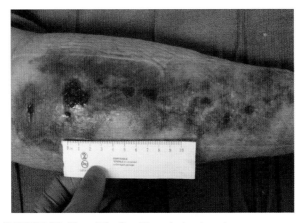

FIGURE 7-22. Vasculitis after 12 weeks treatment.

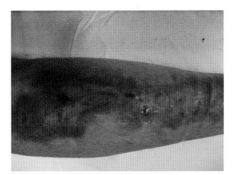

FIGURE 7-23. Full closure after 16 weeks treatment.

Pathophysiology
- Is an autoimmune inflammatory disorder of blood vessels which can result in organ damage, including the skin (see Table 7-4)
- Can be triggered by underlying co-morbidities (e.g. infection, malignancy, connective tissue disorders, hepatitis), termed secondary systemic vasculitis;

or can be idiopathic, termed primary systemic vasculitis;[22] or idiopathic cutaneous leukocytoclastic vasculitis[23]

• Extracellular vesicles (released during programmed cells death) are involved in cell-to-cell communication, including carrying autoantigens, and thereby have an important role in inflammation, autoimmune responses, pro-coagulation, endothelial dysfunction/damage, angiogenesis, and intimal hyperplasia—all histopathological findings in vasculitis[24]

TABLE 7-4. Vasculitic syndromes based upon the affected vessels

Name	Typical Vessels Involved	Symptoms
Churg-Strauss syndrome	Small and medium vessel	Three stages: 1. Airway inflammation, asthma, allergic rhinitis 2. Hypereosinophilia 3. Vasculitis with tissue necrosis
Cryoglobulinemia	Small vessels in the toes and feet	Purpura and Raynaud's phenomenon that progresses to painful skin necrosis and ulceration
Giant cell arteritis	Temporal and cranial arteries	Headaches, temporal pain, visual disturbances, scalp sensitivity, dry cough with respiratory symptoms, fever, upper extremity weakness and sensory changes
Henoch-Schönlein purpura	Small vessels	Purpura, arthritis, abdominal pain (usually in children)
Immune complex-associated vasculitis	Small vessels to neurons	Peripheral neuropathy
Microscopic polyangiitis	Small vessels to organs	Ischemia, hemorrhage, loss of organ function
Polyarteritis nodosa	Small and medium arteries	Subcutaneous nodules or projections of lesions; fever, chills, tachycardia, arthralgia, myositis, motor and sensory neuropathies
Primary angiitis of the CNS	Small and medium vessels in the brain and spinal cord	Brain: headache, altered mental status, focal CNS deficits; spinal cord: lower extremity weakness, bladder dysfunction
Takayasu's arteritis	Aorta, aorta branches, pulmonary arteries	Inflammatory phase with flu-like symptoms, pulseless upper extremity, claudication, renal artery disease
Wegener's granulomatosis (granulomatosis with polyangiitis)	Small and medium vessels	Organ failure (lung and kidneys), variable including skin, depending on the vessels involved

Adapted with permission from Schiffman M, Low M: Chronic Wounds, Wound Dressings and Wound Healing, vol 6. Switzerland; Springer; 2018.

Clinical presentation (dermal only)
- Depends upon the arteries that are inflamed
- Urticaria
- Erythema
- Petechiae
- Purpura, with or without papules
- Hemorrhagic vesicles and bullae
- Nodules
- Livedo reticularis
- Deep-punched out full-thickness wounds
- Skin necrosis
- Exquisite burning pain and deep aching[23]

Medical management
- Treatment of any underlying co-morbidities associated with secondary vasculitis
- Referral to an immunology specialist; treatment of the vasculitis involves high-dose glucocorticoids in conjunction with immune-suppressants for 12 weeks with tapering over 6 months and adjustment to maintain remission[25]

Wound management
- Debride necrotic tissue by enzymatic, autolytic, sharp, or contact low-frequency ultrasound; apply topical lidocaine prior to treatment especially in the early stages
- Apply non-contact low-frequency ultrasound to assist in healing, to reduce inflammation, and to mitigate pain
- Apply antimicrobial, absorbent dressings or non-adherent dressings (e.g. X-Cell, Medline, Mundelein IL) to promote autolytic debridement; cover with silicone-backed foam to avoid painful dressing changes
- Apply compression bandages to lower extremity wounds to manage the edema that accompanies chronic inflammation[26]

CRYOGLOBULINEMIA
Figures 7-24 through 7-27

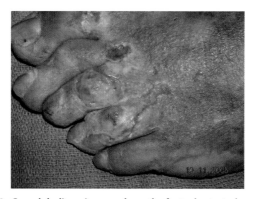

FIGURE 7-24. Cryoglobulinemia wounds on the foot; also tested positive for MRSA.

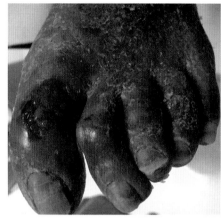

FIGURE 7-25. Cryoglobulinemia wounds after treatment.

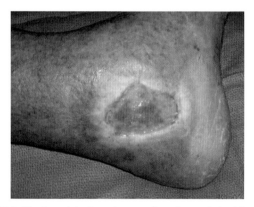

FIGURE 7-26. Cryoglobulinemia wound on the medial ankle.

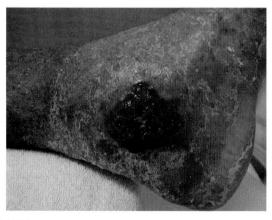

FIGURE 7-27. Cryoglobulinemia wound after treatment.

Pathophysiology
- Abnormal immunoglobulins, termed cryoglobulins, coagulate or become gel-like in the blood when temperatures are below core body temperature (37° C, 99° F).
- Cryoglobulinemia results when these immune complexes precipitate and clog the blood vessels, resulting in vasculitic damage that causes hypoxic skin changes, ischemic wounds, and/or other organ damage.
- Symptoms may be reversible if the environmental temperature is warmed.
- Three types based on the antibody that is produced:
  - Type I—usually with a monoclonal IgM, IgG, or IgA that does not have rheumatic activity; most often related to cancer of the blood or immune system, e.g. multiple myeloma
  - Type II—with polyclonal IgG, monoclonal IgM, and rheumatoid factor activity, also referred to as mixed cryoglobulinemia; most often occurs in people who have an infectious disease, e.g. hepatitis C and HIV, or autoimmune disorders
  - Type III—with polyclonal IgG, polyclonal IgM, and rheumatoid factor activity; also called mixed cryoglobulinemia; associated with other inflammatory disorders, e.g. Sjogren syndrome[27]

> **Diagnostic Clue:** Cryoglobulinemia is a specific type of vasculitis, frequently associated with hepatitis C. It does have some differentiating characteristics, mainly that it exacerbates during cold weather and is sometimes reversible if the environment is warmed. The dermal wounds associated with cryoglobulinemia tend to occur on the distal digits and feet, whereas vasculitis from other pathologies may occur on other anatomical parts.

Clinical presentation (see Table 7-5)
- Systemic signs with Types II and III include difficulty breathing, fatigue, glomerulonephritis, joint pain, muscle pain
- Integumentary signs begin with purpura and Raynaud's phenomenon and progress to skin necrosis and ulceration
- Meltzer triad associated with types II and III includes arthralgia, purpura, and weakness.

Medical management
- Treat any underlying diseases associated with all types
- Advise patient to avoid cold temperatures and to keep extremities warm, especially with integumentary changes on the distal digits
- Refer to rheumatologist for treatment which involves the use of glucocorticoids, immunosuppressants, interferon, cytotoxic medications, and plasmapheresis, as well as specific combinations, depending upon the type, severity, and underlying disorders[28]

Wound management
- Antimicrobial dressings to treat and/or prevent infection
- Dressings (e.g. X-Cell, Medline, Mundelein IL, and petrolatum gauze) to promote autolytic debridement of necrotic tissue and help mitigate pain with dressing changes

TABLE 7-5.   Symptoms of cryoglobulinemia

Local/Integumentary	General/Systemic
Type I	Type I
Lesions in head and mucosa	Retinal hemorrhage
Acrocyanosis	Arterial thrombosis
Severe Raynaud's phenomenon	Renal disease
Digital ulceration	Types II and III
Skin necrosis	Breathing difficulty
Livedo reticularis	Fatigue
Purpura	Arthralgia (PIP, MCP, knees, ankles)
Types II and III	Myalgia
Lesions in lower extremities	Immune complex deposition
Erythematous macules	Cough
Palpable purpura	Pleurisy
Raynaud phenomenon	Abdominal pain
Cutaneous vasculitis	Fever
Peripheral neuropathy	Hepatomegaly or signs of cirrhosis
Nailfold capillary abnormalities	Hypertension

Data from Edgerton CC, Diamond HS. Cryoglobulinemia Clinical Presentation. Medscape; January 9, 2019.

- Topical anesthetics prior to treatment due to intense ischemic pain
- Modified compression (e.g. with short stretch bandages) to manage edema that occurs with chronic inflammation and to help keep extremities warm
- Educate patient on strategies to keep extremities warm in order to help prevent recurrence[26]

PYODERMA GANGRENOSUM
Figures 7-28 and 7-29

Pathophysiology
- A chronic, autoimmune disorder of unknown etiology that leads to painful skin necrosis
- A rapidly evolving condition often associated with other inflammatory diseases (e.g. Crohn's disease, inflammatory bowel syndrome, arthritis), hematologic malignancies,[29] or severe trauma (e.g. surgery)[30,31]
- A poorly understood disorder that is usually a diagnosis of exclusion thought to be caused by up-regulation and aberrant trafficking of polymorphonuclear neutrophils (PMNs) with subsequent release of PMN-stimulating cytokines

Clinical presentation
- Usually occurs on the lower extremities or trunk[31]
- Begins as a tender nodule or pustule that progresses to an open lesion[30]
- Presents with a raised, violaceous, undermined border and a cribriform base[31]
- Often accompanied with fever and malaise
- Is accompanied by intense, disproportional pain
- Includes common abnormal laboratory values such as leukocytosis, elevated erythrocyte sedimentation rate, and elevated C-reactive protein

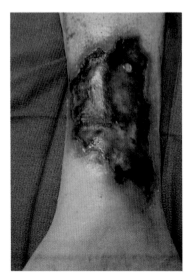

FIGURE 7-28. Pyoderma gangrenosum on the lower extremity.

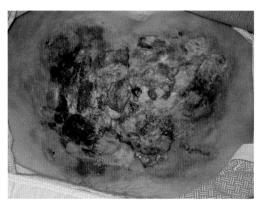

FIGURE 7-29. Pyoderma gangrenosum on the abdomen of a female with diabetes, after she had a hysterectomy.

Medical management
- Treatment of any underlying disorders
- Rule out infection by performing biopsy from the wound border including subcutaneous tissue
- Avoidance of debridement of necrotic tissue; this may lead to pathergy or exacerbation of the skin lesion due to added trauma
- Administration of systemic steroids and cyclosporine,[30] and antibiotics when indicated
- Use of tumor necrosis factor alpha antagonists (infliximab and adalimumab) when traditional treatment fails[31]

> **Diagnostic Clue:** The biopsy from the erythematous skin adjacent to the ulcer may reveal both superficial and deep vascular injury with skin and subcutaneous necrosis and a dense lymphocytic infiltrate.[32]

Wound management
- Avoid aggressive debridement; remove only loose detached eschar that shows signs of re-epithelialization beneath it
- Cover lesions with non-adherent mesh or silicone-backed wicking foam that allows the drainage to escape to a secondary dressing, thereby alleviating some of the pain associated with dressing changes

ANTIPHOSPHOLIPID SYNDROME

Figures 7-30 through 7-32

Pathophysiology
- Is an acquired autoimmune systemic disorder in which antibodies are directed against one or more phospholipid-binding proteins (anti-ß2-glycoprotein 1, moderately-high titer anticardiolipin, or lupus anticoagulant) or their associated proteins[33]
- Results in hyper-coagulation within the microvasculature with subsequent tissue death
- Occurs with or without associated rheumatic disease (e.g. systemic lupus erythematosus)
- In some cases, it causes obstetrical events, defined as early preeclampsia which is unexplained fetal death at >10 weeks gestation; or ≥3 spontaneous abortions at <10 weeks gestation.[34]
- At risk patients are listed in Table 7-6.

Clinical presentation
- Dermal signs (livedo reticularis, cutaneous ulcerations, livedoid vasculopathy, Raynaud phenomenon, pyoderma gangrenosum-like ulcers, nail fold ulcers, digital ischemia, splinter hemorrhages, widespread cutaneous necrosis, pseudo-Kaposi sarcoma, superficial thrombophlebitis migrans) in ≤70% of cases[34]
- Systemic complications—thrombocytopenia, hemolytic anemia, valvular heart disease, nephropathy

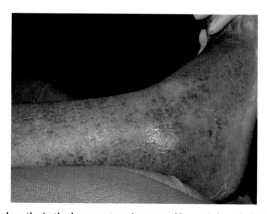

FIGURE 7-30. Vasculopathy in the lower extremity caused by antiphospholipid syndrome.

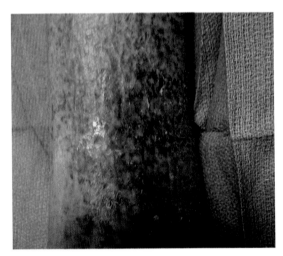

FIGURE 7-31. Hyper-coagulation visible in the lower extremity caused by antiphospholipid syndrome.

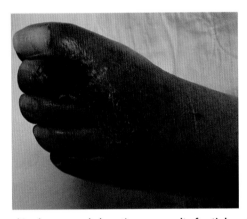

FIGURE 7-32. Forefoot skin changes and ulceration as a result of antiphospholipid syndrome.

Medical management
- Prophylactic
  - Eliminate risk factors (oral contraceptives, smoking, hypertension, hyperlipidemia)
  - For patients with SLE, consider hydroxychloroquine
  - For patients with hyperlipidemia, consider statins
- Treatment of thrombosis
  - Anticoagulation with IV or subcutaneous heparin, followed by warfarin therapy
  - INR for venous thrombosis—2.0–3.0; for arterial thrombosis—3.0; for recurrent thrombotic events—3.0–4.0
  - Rituximab for patients with recurrent thrombosis despite adequate anticoagulation
- Treatment of obstetric patients
  - Prophylactic anticoagulation (with subcutaneous heparin and low-dose aspirin) during pregnancy and for 6 weeks post-partum for women with APS and who have a history of thrombosis[35]

TABLE 7-6. Patients at risk for developing antiphospholipid syndrome

Other autoimmune or rheumatic diseases associated with APS
• Systemic lupus erythematosus
• Sjogren syndrome
• Rheumatoid arthritis
• Autoimmune thrombocytopenic purpura
• Autoimmune hemolytic anemia
• Psoriatic arthritis
• Systemic sclerosis
• Mixed connective-tissue disease
• Polymyalgia rheumatica or giant cell arteritis
• Behcet's syndrome
Infections associated with APS
• Syphilis
• Hepatitis C
• HIV infection
• Human T-cell lymphotrophic virus type 1 infection
• Malaria
• Bacterial septicemia
Drugs associated with APS
• Cardiac—Procainamide, quinidine, propranolol, hydralazine
• Neuroleptic or psychiatric—Phenytoin, chlorpromazine
• Other—Interferon alfa, quinine, amoxicillin

Data from Movva S, Diamond HS, Belilos E, et al: Antiphospholipid Syndrome Clinical Presentation. https://emedicine.medscape.com.

Wound management
- Conservative wound care for skin lesions
- Recognition of slow healing for wounds caused by other etiologies on patients with APS

PEMPHIGUS
Figures 7-33 through 7-37

Pathophysiology
- Is an autoimmune blistering disease that affects the skin and mucous membranes
- Typically occurs between 40 and 60 years of age
- Occurs when autoantibodies attack desmoglein, the "glue" or adhesion molecule at the desmosomal cell junction in the suprabasal layer of the epidermis, resulting in the destruction of the adhesion molecules (termed acantholysis) and thereby initiating an inflammatory response that causes the blistering
- Blister sloughing that can cause open wounds with a propensity for infection
- Has four distinct types based on the desmogleins that are affected
  - Pemphigus vulgaris—autoantibodies attack desmoglein 3 or desmoglein 1 and 3; is the most common type and affects both skin and mucous membranes; has primary cell adhesion loss in the deeper suprabasal layer

- ○ Pemphigus foliaceous—autoantibodies attack desmoglein 1; affects only the skin in the more superficial epidermis, and is thus milder
- ○ IgA pemphigus vegetans—autoantibodies attack desmoglein 1; forms grouped clusters with crusts in the epidermis
- ○ Paraneoplastic pemphigus—autoantibodies attack plakins and desmogleins and weaken cell adhesion; inflammatory cells infiltrate the skin, thereby damaging the structure of the adjacent cells; is associated with underlying malignancies; e.g. lymphoma[36]

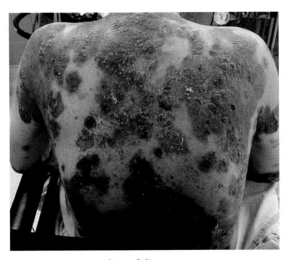

FIGURE 7-33. Pemphigus foliaceous.

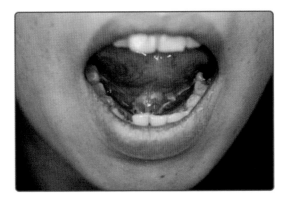

FIGURE 7-34. Pemphigus vulgaris.

Reproduced with permission from Hashimoto T, Teye K, Ishii N. Clinical and immu-nological studies of 49 cases of various types of intercellular IgA dermatosis and 13 cases of classical subcorneal pustular dermatosis examined at Kurume University, Br J Dermatol 2017 Jan;176(1):168-175.

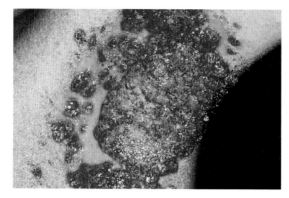

FIGURE 7-35. IgA pemphigus vegetans.

Reproduced with permission from Weston WL, Friednash M, Hashimoto T, Seline P, Huff JC, Morelli JG. A novel childhood pemphigus vegetans variant of intraepidermal neutrophilic IgA dermatosis, J Am Acad Dermatol 1998 Apr;38(4):635-638.

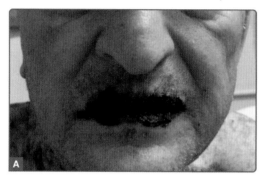

FIGURE 7-36. Paraneoplastic pemphigus lesions on the mouth.

Reproduced with permission from Kang S, Amagai M, Bruckner AL, et al: Fitzpatrick's Dermatology, 9th ed. New York, NY: McGraw Hill; 2019.

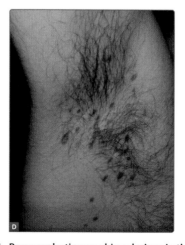

FIGURE 7-37. Paraneoplastic pemphigus lesions in the axilla.

Reproduced with permission from Kang S, Amagai M, Bruckner AL, et al: Fitzpatrick's Dermatology, 9th ed. New York, NY: McGraw Hill; 2019.

Clinical presentation
- Pemphigus vulgaris
  - Involves mucosa and skin, especially scalp, face, axilla, groin, trunk, points of pressure
  - Has painful oral mucosal erosions
  - Presents with flaccid blisters, erosions, crusts, and macular erythema in areas of skin involvement
- Pemphigus foliaceous
  - Affects face and chest
  - Presents with flaccid blisters, erosions, crusts
  - Leaves hyperpigmentation with healing
- IgA pemphigus
  - Pruritus
  - Vesicles, pustules, and circinate plaques[37]
- Paraneoplastic pemphigus
  - Occurs exclusively with a malignancy, usually a lymphoproliferative disorder
  - Presents consistently with severe stomatitis resulting in lesions of the mouth
  - Has high mortality rate[38]

Medical management
- Confirm diagnosis with immunofluorescence to demonstrate IgG antibodies against the cell surface of intra-epidermal keratinocytes
- Oral corticosteroids until lesions resolve (prednisone/rituximab)
- IV immunoglobulin for cases when prednisone/rituximab does not eliminate circulating autoantibodies[39]
- Maintenance doses of corticosteroids to prevent recurrence

Wound management
- Intra-lesional injections or topical application of corticosteroids
- Antimicrobial dressings over denuded areas to help prevent infection
- Hydrotherapy when the disease is widespread and in the crusty phase
- Secondary dressings (e.g. silicone-backed foam without adhesive borders) anchored with surgical or fish-net garments[26]

PEMPHIGOID

Figures 7-38 and 7-39

Pathophysiology
- Typically occurs in the elderly (>65 years)
- Is a sub-epidermal autoimmune disease that affects primarily the skin
- Autoantibodies are directed against BP antigen 180 and BP antigen 230, both components of the hemidesmosones in the basal layer of the epidermis
- An inflammatory response results in infiltration of lymphocytes, histiocytes, and eosinophils which release proteases that degrade hemidesmosone proteins with subsequent loss of anchoring filaments, followed by blistering[40]
- Heals without scarring[36]
- Has two types
  - Bullous pemphigoid—occurs on the skin
  - Mucous membrane pemphigoid—occurs on the mucous membrane, most frequently of the eyes and mouth

Clinical presentation (bullous pemphigoid)

- Occurs on the inner thighs, lower abdomen, axilla, and flexor surfaces of the extremities
- Presents as itching that progresses to urticarial lesions, erythematous edema, papules, eczematous lesions, and widespread tense bullae filled with clear fluid[26,37]
- Tends to persist for months or years with spontaneous remission and flare-ups

Medical management

- Direct immunofluorescence studies on the normal-appearing perilesional skin, and if positive, follow with indirect immunofluorescence studies of the serum[40]
- Anti-inflammatory agents (dapsone, corticosteroids, tetracyclines)
- Immunosuppressant agents (azathioprine, methotrexate, mycophenolate mofetil, cyclophosphamide)[40]
- Treatment for 6–60 months, with no maintenance therapy required

Wound management

- Antimicrobial non-adherent dressings over any open areas due to denuded blisters in order to prevent infection and promote re-epithelialization, as well as to minimize pain during dressing changes

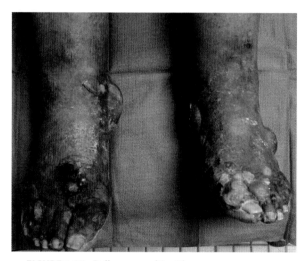

FIGURE 7-38. Bullous pemphigoid.

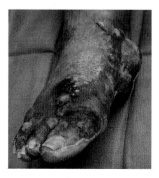

FIGURE 7-39. Bullous pemphigoid.

SCLERODERMA

Figures 7-40 through 7-42

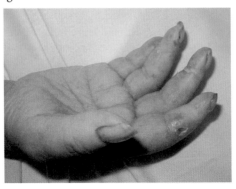

FIGURE 7-40. Scleroderma wound on the hand.

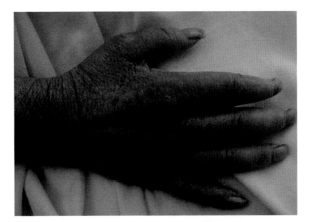

FIGURE 7-41. Tapered fingers characteristic of scleroderma.

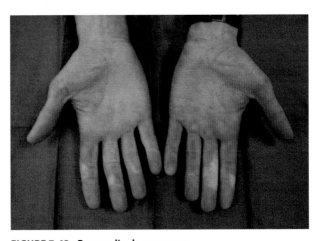

FIGURE 7-42. Raynaud's phenomenon.

Pathophysiology
- Is a group of autoimmune diseases that result in extensive scarring and disfigurement as it progresses
- Causes skin to become thick and hard (sclerotic) with an accumulation of scar tissue, resulting in loss of skin elasticity, joint range of motion, muscle strength, mobility, and function
- Also causes damage to internal organs (heart, blood vessels, lungs, esophagus, kidneys), a major predictor of prognosis for each patient
- Involves the following sequence: arteriole endothelial cells die by apoptosis and are replaced by collagen; inflammatory cells infiltrate the arteriole and cause more damage by up-regulation of adhesion molecules and chemokines; activation of fibroblasts and myofibroblasts leads to production of excessive collagen, decreased extracellular matrix degradation, and thereby the scarred fibrotic tissue[41,42]

Clinical presentation
Clinical signs and symptoms have been categorized into the following types of scleroderma:
- Localized—affects only the skin, not the internal organs
  - Morphea—causes discolored patches on the skin
  - Linear—causes streaks or bands of thick hard skin on the arms and legs
- Systemic
  - Diffuse—progresses rapidly, affects large areas of the skin and one or more organs
  - Limited—affects only the arms, face, and hands
    - CREST: See Table 7-7 for symptoms
    - Sine scleroderma includes Raynaud phenomenon and internal involvement without sclerotic skin[43]

Medical management
- Referral to a rheumatologist for appropriate medications, especially in severe cases
- Vasodilators for treatment of Raynaud's phenomenon
- Immuno-suppressants (e.g. methotrexate and cyclosporine) for systemic types
- Educate patients to preserve skin integrity with protective strategies, e.g. wearing gloves when doing housework, avoiding caustic liquids, wearing thermal socks and gloves in colder weather to avoid Raynaud's phenomenon, using moisturizers to avoid dry skin[26]
- Referral to a hand surgeon for disabling hand deformities[44]
- Referral to a pedorthotist for adaptive shoes in the case of foot deformities that affect patient's ability to ambulate

TABLE 7-7. Symptoms of CREST, a limited systemic scleroderma syndrome

Calcinosis—calcium deposits, usually in the fingers
Raynaud phenomenon—color changes in fingers and sometimes toes after exposure to cold temperatures
Esophageal dysfunction—loss of muscle control which can cause difficulty swallowing
Sclerodactyly—tapering deformity of the bones of the fingers
Telangiectasia—small red spots on the skin of the fingers, face, or inside of the mouth

Wound management
- Enzymatic debridement with collagenase for necrotic tissue
- Occlusive dressings to assist with autolytic debridement
- Non-adherent dressings to minimize pain and avoid tearing the skin upon removal
- Apply topical anesthetics 15–20 minutes prior to treatment of painful wounds[26]

NECROBIOSIS LIPOIDICA (NL)

Figures 7-43 through 7-45

Pathophysiology
- Is a rare idiopathic granulomatous disease of collagen degeneration with risk of ulceration[45]
- Involves the dermis and sometimes the subcutaneous fat layer
- May be associated with pre-diabetes or diabetes; however, not all patients with necrobiosis lipoidica have diabetes[46]
- Causes thickening of the blood vessel walls and fat deposition, thus making the integumentary symptoms similar to vasculitis
- Has unknown etiology; however, has three suggested theories of pathogenesis:
  - T cell mediated hypersensitivity reaction
  - Immune-mediated vasculopathy
  - Primary degenerative disorder of the dermal collagen[46]

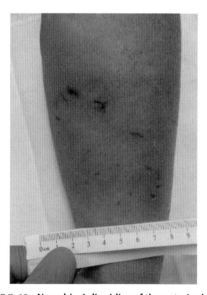

FIGURE 7-43. Necrobiosis lipoidica of the anterior lower leg.

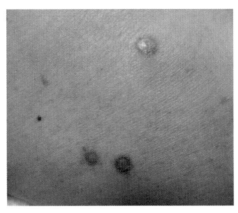

FIGURE 7-44. Annular lesions typical of NL lesions.

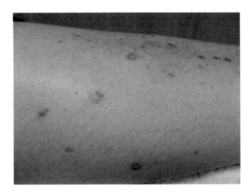

FIGURE 7-45. Hyperpigmented scarring typical of NL healed lesions.

Clinical presentation
- Usually presents on the lower extremities, in females more than males
- Is bilateral but asymmetric on the tibial surface
- Begins as a rash or 1-3 mm slightly raised spots
- Progresses to irregular ovoid reddish-brown plaques with shiny yellow centers and violaceous indurated borders
- Has good granulation in the wound bed but no epithelial migration
- Presents with pain and edema
- Remodels with residual round patches of hyperpigmentation[26]

Medical management
- Confirm diagnosis with histopathology; biopsy shows horizontal granulomatous inflammation in the dermis, composed of layers of histiocytes and multinucleated giant cells with intervening layers of inflammatory infiltrate containing lymphocytes, plasma cells, and eosinophils
- Treat mild to moderate cases with topical or intralesional steroids
- Treat with a combination of pentoxifylline, hydroxychloroquine, and topical clobetasol[47]

Wound management
- 0.1% topical tacrolimus ointment
- Collagen matrix dressings
- Phototherapy (Psoralen plus ultraviolet A)[46]
- Low-frequency non-contact ultrasound to mitigate pain
- Non-adherent saline-impregnated cellulose dressings (X-Cell, Medline, Mundelein IL) to promote autolytic debridement and reduce pain with dressing changes
- Multi-layer compression wraps to reduce lower extremity edema[26]

HIDRADENITIS SUPPURATIVA

Figures 7-46 through 7-49

Pathophysiology
- Is a chronic inflammatory skin disorder that affects the hair follicles in intertriginous regions (inguinal, axillary, inframammary, genital, perineal, and perianal areas)
- Is a follicular occlusion disorder, leading to the release of pro-inflammatory cytokines such as IL-1ß,IL-12, IL-23, and TNF-α[48]
- Involves the over-activation of the innate immune system[49]
- Begins as an occlusive plug that forms inside the hair follicle which causes further accumulation of infiltrates, eventually resulting in the release of destructive pro-inflammatory cytokines into the surrounding skin, thereby causing a severe inflammatory response[49]
- Occurs most frequently in females, with the average age of onset between 20 and 40, after puberty; symptoms may be aggravated with the onset of menstruation[49]

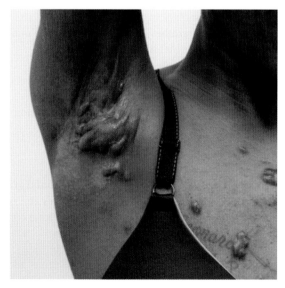

FIGURE 7-46. Stage 1 Hidradenitis suppurativa.

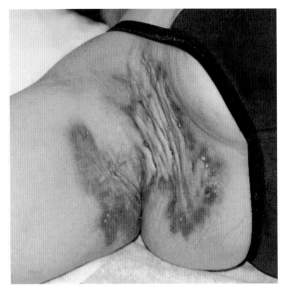

FIGURE 7-47. Stage 2 Hidradenitis suppurativa.

- Common co-morbidities include obesity, metabolic syndrome, cardiovascular risk factors, endocrine co-morbidities (hormone dysfunction, thyroid dysfunction), gastrointestinal disorders, rheumatic disease, and psychiatric disorders as a result of the chronic pain and physical limitations[48]
- Risk factors include family history of the disorder, smoking, and obesity

Clinical presentation
- Initial symptoms include deep-seated inflamed, pea-sized nodules at the site of hair follicles, progressing to infected, painful wounds with exudate and odor due to infection, as well as sinus tracts that become infected and exhibit biofilm[49]
- As lesions heal, they become fibrotic, causing disfiguring scars with tight skin and possible limited range of motion[50]
- The Hurley staging system is used to categorize symptoms into the following three stages:
  - Stage 1: abscess formation (single or multiple) without sinus tracts and scarring
  - Stage 2: recurrent abscesses with sinus tracts and scarring; rare remissions
  - Stage 3: diffuse areas of involvement across a broad area of the body characterized by scarring and oozing lesions[51]

Medical management
- Stage 1
  - Topical clindamycin (1% solution)
  - Intralesional corticosteroids (e.g. 10 mg/mL triamcinolone)
  - Punch debridement of new lesions to prevent progression to an abscess or sinus tract
  - Topical 15% resorcinol to reduce pain and lesion size[51]

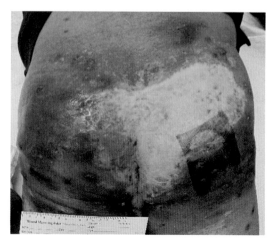

FIGURE 7-48. Stage 3 Hidradenitis suppurativa.

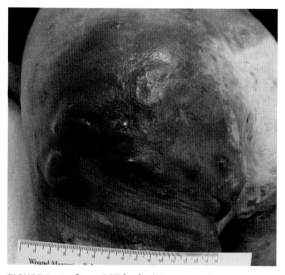

FIGURE 7-49. Stage 3 Hidradenitis suppurativa.

- Stage 2
  - Systemic antibiotics (e.g. oral tetracycline, erythromycin, minocycline, doxycycline)[49]
  - Combination of clindamycin and rifampin
  - Dapsone
  - Oral retinoids
  - Hormonal therapy (cyproterone, alone or with oral contraceptives for women who are not pregnant)
  - Surgical excision for those who do not respond to conservative treatment[51]
- Stage 3
  - TNF-α inhibitors (adalimumab, infliximab)

- Biologic therapies (ustekinumab, anakinra, canakinumab, MABp1); relapse is common if treatment is discontinued[51]
  - Referral to a plastic surgeon for surgical excision and skin grafting
- General suggestions
  - Early intervention for optimal results and to prevent progression
  - Good local hygiene with soap
  - Weight reduction
  - Smoking cessation[52]
  - Wearing loose fitting clothing to avoid friction and pressure[50]
  - Biopsy of long-standing lesions that may develop squamous cell carcinoma[53]

Wound management
- Topical antimicrobial, absorbent dressings
- De-roofing of lesions, followed by probing to locate sinus tracts
- Pulsed lavage with suction using a tracking tip at low psi, followed by filling the track with antimicrobial alginate, cadexomer iodine, or foam dressings (ones that can be removed without leaving fibers in the sinus)
- Secondary dressings of non-adherent materials (e.g. silicone-backed foam)
- Negative pressure wound therapy on larger lesions and sinuses
- Charcoal dressings to help decrease odor[53]

REFERENCES

1. Luttrell T. Healing response in acute and chronic wounds. In Hamm R, ed. *Text and Atlas of Wound Diagnosis and Treatment.* New York, NY: McGraw Hill Education. 2019;15-66.
2. Davis D. *The Beautiful Cure: The Revolution in Immunology and What It Means to Your Health.* Chicago, IL: The University of Chicago Press.
3. Alinaghi F, Bennike NH, Egeberg A, Thyssen JP, Johansen JD. Prevalence of contact allergy in the general population: A systematic review and meta-analysis. *Contact Dermatitis.* 2019;80(2):77-85.
4. Bonitsis NG, Tatsioni A, Bassioukas K, Ioannidis JP. Allergens responsible for allergic contact dermatitis among children: A systematic review and meta-analysis. *Contact Dermatitis.* 2011;64(5):245-257.
5. Nassau S, Fonacier L. Allergic contact dermatitis. *Med Clin N Am.* 2019;104:61-76. Available at https://doi.org/10.1016/j.mcna.2019.08.012. Accessed March 10, 2020.
6. Milani EC, Cohen DE. Contact dermatitis. *Dermatol Clin.* 37 (2019);21–28. Available at https://doi.org/1016/j.det.2018.07.005. Accessed March 10, 2020.
7. Frempah B, Luckett-Chastain LR, Calhous KN, Gallucci RM. Keratinocyte-specific deletion of the IL-6RA exacerbates the inflammatory response during irritant contact dermatitis. *Toxicology.* 2019;423(7):123-131.
8. Saary J, Qureshi R, Palda V, DeKoven J, Pratt M, Skotnicki-Grant S, et.al. A systematic review of contact dermatitis treatment and prevention. *J Am Acad Dermatol.* 2005;53(5):845.
9. Al-Otaibi ST, Alqahtani HAM. Management of contact dermatitis. *J Dermatol Surg.* 2015;19(2):86-91.
10. Shiohara T, Mizukawa Y. Drug-induced hypersensitivity syndrome (DiHS)/drug reaction with eosinophilia and systemic symptoms (DRESS): An update in 2019. *Allergology International.* 2019;68:301-308.
11. Oussalah A, Ypi V, Mayorga C, Blanca M, Barbaud A, Nakonechna A, et al. Genetic variants associated with T-cell medicated cutaneous adverse drug reactions: A PRISMA-compliant

systematic review – an EAACI Position Paper. *Allergy.* 2020 Jan 3. Doi:10.1111/all.14174. Accessed March 13, 2020.

12. Jarjour S, Barrette M, Normand V, Rouleau JL, Dube MP, de Denus S. Genetic markers associated with cutaneous adverse drug reactions to allopurinol: A systematic review. *Pharmacogenomics.* 2015;16(7):755-767.

13. Tangamomsukan W, Lohitnavy M. Association between HLA-B*1301 and dapsone-induced cutaneous adverse drug reactions: A systematic review and meta-analysis. *JAMA Dermatol.* 2018;154(4):441-446.

14. Damiani G, Eggenhoffner R, Pigatto PDM, Bragazzi NL. Nanotechnology meets atopic dermatitis: Current solutions, challenges and future prospects. Insights and implications from a systematic review of the literature. *Bioactive Materials.* 2019;4:380-386.

15. Saini S, Pansare M. New insights and treatments in atopic dermatitis. *Pediatr Clin N Am.* 2019;66:1021-1033.

16. Chan S, Cornelius V, Cro S, Harper JI, Lack G. Treatment effect of omalizumab on severe pediatric atopic dermatitis: The ADAPT randomized clinical trial. *JAMA Pediatr.* 2019;11. Doi: 10.1001/jamapediatrics.2019.4476. Accessed March 11, 2020.

17. Guttman-Yassky E, Thaci D, Pangan AL, Hong HC, Papp KA, Reich K, et al. Upadacitinib in adults with moderate to severe atopic dermatitis: 16-week results from a randomized, placebo-controlled trial. *J Allergy Clin Immunol.* 2020;145(3):877-884.

18. Youssef R, Hafez V, Elkholy Y, Mourad A. Glycerol 85% efficacy on atopic skin and its microbiome: A randomized controlled trial with clinical and bacteriological evaluation. *J Dermatolog Treat.* 2020. doi: 10.1080/09546634.2019.1708246. Accessed March 11, 2020.

19. Woo TE, Sibley CD. The emerging utility of the cutaneous microbiome in the treatment of acne and atopic dermatitis. *J Am Acad Derm.* September 6, 2019. Available at https://doi.org/10.1016/j.jaad.2019.08.078. Accessed March 12, 2020.

20. https://www.mayoclinic.org/diseases-conditions/atopic-dermatitis-eczema/diagnosis-treatment/drc-20353279. Accessed March 12, 2020.

21. Cardona ID, Kempe EE, Lary C, Ginder JH, Jain N. Frequent versus infrequent bathing in pediatric atopic dermatitis: A randomized clinical trial. *J Allergy and Clin Immunol.* 2020;8(3):1014-1021.

22. Gwaltney KG, Tracy JA. Peripheral nerve vasculitis. *Neurologic Clinics.* 2019;37(2):303–333.

23. Younger D, Carlson A. Dermatologic aspects of systemic vasculitis. *Neurologic Clinics.* 2019;37(2):465-473.

24. Wu X, Liu Y, Wei W, Liu M. Extracellular vesicles in autoimmune vasculitis – little dirts light the fire in blood vessels. *Autoimmunity Reviews.* 2019;18(6):593-606.

25. Ntatsake E, Carruthers D, Chakravarty K, et al. BSR and BHPR guideline for the management of adults with ANCA-associated vasculitis. *Rheumatology.* 2014;53(12):2306-2309.

26. Hamm R, Shah JB. Atypical wounds. In Hamm R, ed. *Text and Atlas of Wound Diagnosis and Treatment.* New York, NY: McGraw Hill Education. 2019;235-268.

27. Cryoglobulinemia. Available at https://en.wikipedia.org/wiki/Cryoglobulinemia. Accessed March 20, 2020.

28. Ostojic P, Jeremic IR. Managing refractory cryoglobulinemic vasculitis: Challenges and solutions. *J Inflamm Res.* 2017;10(5):49-54.

29. Montagnon CM, Fracica EA, Patel AA, Camilleri MJ, Murad MH, Dingli D, et al. Pyoderma gangrenosum in hematolgic malignancies: A systematic review. *J Am Acad Dermatol.* 2019. Available at https://doi.org/10.1016/j.jaad.2019.09.032. Accessed March 16, 2020.

30. Murata T, Kyozuka H, Fukuda T, Hiraiwa T, Yamaguchi A, Fujimori K. Incisional pyoderma gangrenosum after caesarean section: Two case reports. *Case Reports in Women's Health.* 2019;23:e00128.

31. Almukhtar R, Armenta AM, Martin J, Goodwin BP, Vincent B, Lee B. Dacso MM. Delayed diagnosis of post-surgical pyoderma gangrenosum: A multicenter case series and review of literature. *International Journal of Surgery Case Reports.* 2018;44:152-156.
32. Su WP, et al. Pyoderma gangrenosum: Clinicopathologic correlation and proposed diagnositic criteria. *Int J Dermatol.* 2004;43(11):790-800.
33. Sammaritano L. Antiphopholipid syndrome. *Best Practive & Research Clinical Rheumatology.* 2019. Available at https://doi.org/10.1016/j.berh.2019.101463. Accessed March 18, 2020.
34. Zhang Y, Riddle ND, Seminario-Vidal L. Post-partum cutaneous manifestation of antiphospholipid syndrome. *Human Pathology: Case Reports.* Available at https://org/10.1016/j.ehpc.2019.200334. Accessed March 18, 2020.
35. Movva S, Diamond HS, Belilos E, Carsons S. Antiphospholipid syndrome clinical presentation. Updated September 30, 2018. Available at https://emedicine.medscape.com/article/333221. Accessed March 18, 2020.
36. Available at http://www.pemphigus.org/living-with-pemphigus-pemphigoid/all-about-pemphigus-patient-edition. Accessed March 19, 2020.
37. Kridin K, Papel PM, Jones VA, Cordova A, Amber KT. IgA pemphigus: A systematic review. Journal *of the American Academy of dermatology.* 2019. Available at https://doi.org/10.1016/j.jaad.2019.11.059. Accessed March 19, 2020.
38. Anhalt GJ, Mimouni D. Paraneoplastic pemphigus. In: Wolff K, ed. *Fitzpatrick's Dermatology in General Medicine.* 8th ed. New York, NY: McGraw-Hill. 2012;Chapter 55.
39. Grando SA, Rigas M, Chernyavsky A. Rationale for including intravenous immunoglobulin in the multidrug protocol of curative treatment of pemphigus vulgaris and development of an assay predicting disease relapse. *International Immunopharmacology.* 2020;82. Available at https://doi.org/10.1016/j.intimp.2020.106385. Accessed March 19, 2020.
40. Chan LS. Bullous pemphigoid. 2018. Available at https://emedicine.medscape.com/article/1062391-overview#a6. Accessed March 19, 2020.
41. Gabrielli A, Avvedimento EV, Krieg T. Scleroderma. *N Engl J Med.* 2009;360;1989-2003.
42. Tsou PS, Sawalha AH. Unfolding the pathogenesis of scleroderma through genomics and epigenomics. *J Autoimmun.* 2017;83:73-94.
43. Furst EA. Scleroderma: A fascinating, troubling disease. *Topics Adv Pract Nursing eJournal.* 2004;4(2). Available at http://www.medscape.com/viewarticle/473349. Accessed August 2, 1918.
44. Williams AA, Hannah MC, Lifchez SD. The scleroderma hand: Manifestations of disease and approach to management. *J Hand Surgery.* 2018;43(6):550-557.
45. Sibbald C, Reid S, Alavi A. Necrobiosis lipoidica. *Dermatol Clin.* 2015;33:343-360.
46. DiCaudo, DL. Necrobiosis Lipoidica (Necrobiosis Lipoidica Diabeticorum). Available at https://www.dermatologyadvisor.com/home/decision-support-in-medicine/dermatology/necrobiosis-lipoidica-necrobiosis-lipoidica-diabeticorum/. Accessed April 8, 2020.
47. Hashemi DA, Nelson CA, Elenitsas R, Rosenbach M. An atypical case of popular necrobiosis lipoidica masquerading as sarcoidosis. *JAAD Case Reports.* 2018;4(8):802-804.
48. Cartron A, Driscoll MS. Comorbidities of hidradenitis suppurativa: A review of the literature. *Int J Women's Dermatol.* 2019;5:330-334.
49. Ead JK, Snyder RJ, Wise J, Cuffy C, Hamed J, Fischborn K. Is PASH syndrome a biofilm disease?: A case series and review of the literature. *Wounds.* 2018;30(8):216–223.
50. Beshara MA. Hidradenitis suppurativa: A clinician's tool for early diagnosis and treatment. *Advances in Skin & Wound Care.* 2010;23(7):328–334.
51. Hurley HJ. Axillary hyperhidrosis, apocrine bromhidrosis, hidradenitis suppurativa, and familial benign pemphigus: surgical approach. In Roenigk RK, Roenigk HH, eds. *Dermatologic Surgery.* New York, NY: Dekker. 1989;729.

52. Nesbitt E, Clements S, Driscoll M. A concise clinician's guide to therapy for hidradenitis suppurativa. *Int J Women's Dermatol.* 2019. Available at https://doi.org/10.1016/j.ijwd.2019.11.004. Accessed March 22, 2020.
53. Oranges T, Janwska A, Chiricozzi A, Romanelli M, Dini V. HS-TIME: A modified TIME concept in hidradenitis suppurativa topical management. *Wounds.* 2019;31(9):222-227.

8

Infected Wounds

INTRODUCTION

Any wound can become infected, and some infections can compromise the integumentary tissue to the extent that they cause wounds. The purpose of this chapter is to give the clinician guidelines as to when and if a wound is infected, as well as to discuss diseases that can cause skin changes and/or open wounds.

Every wound has flora on its surface, and whether or not the wound becomes infected, as well as the resulting impairment of the wound healing process, depends upon both the type of microbe present and the host immune system. Table 8-1 defines the terms used to describe the presence of bacteria on the wound surface and Table 8-2 lists the microorganisms that are most commonly present in chronic wounds. Gram-positive organisms may be the first to invade the chronic wound, followed by gram-negative bacteria, and then anaerobes.[1] Bacterial testing via tissue biopsies or swabs using the Levine method are helpful to determine the number of colony forming units present, as well as antimicrobial sensitivity for antibiotic selection; however, the differential diagnosis of local, superficial critical colonization versus deep chronic wound infection invading the surrounding tissue can be made clinically based on the following signs and symptoms:

- Critical colonization will have three or more of these signs
  - Static size as measured by length × width over a 2–4 week period
  - Increased amount of exudate
  - Red friable granulation tissue on the wound surface
  - Debris or dead cells on the wound surface
  - Odor that indicates presence of gram-negative or anaerobic organisms
- Infected wounds will have any three of these signs
  - Increased size as measured by length × width
  - Increased temperature of 3°F or more as compared with same place on the opposite limb
  - Bone either exposed or detected with direct probing using a metal instrument
  - New areas of skin breakdown around the wound margin
  - Increased amount of exudate
  - Erythema and/or edema (usually a sign of cellulitis)
  - Odor emanating from the wound after cleansing[2]

TABLE 8-1.   Terms defining the presence of bacteria on a wound

Term	Definition
Contamination	Presence of non-replicating bacteria on the wound surface without any effect upon the wound healing process
Colonization	Presence of replicating bacteria attached to the wound surface with no harm to the host and no effect on the wound healing process
Critical colonization	Presence of replicating bacteria on the wound surface with sufficient numbers to initiate the host immune response and to visibly affect the wound healing process; e.g. the wound size is not decreasing
Infection	Presence of replicating bacteria that have invaded the surrounding tissue with visible effects in the wound healing process and in the periwound tissues as a result of the associated host inflammatory response
Sepsis	Presence of replicating bacteria that produce a whole-body inflammatory state termed systemic inflammatory response syndrome (SIRS)

TABLE 8-2.   Microorganisms most commonly present on chronic wounds

Aerobes
- Acinetobacter baumannii
- Coliforms
- Enterococcus faecalis
- Methicillin-resistant Staphylococcus aureus
- Pseudomonas aeruginosa
- Staphylococcus aureus
- Staphylococcus epidermidis
- Streptococcus pyogenes

Anaerobes
- Bacteroides spp*
- Fusobacterium spp
- Peptostreptococcus spp
- Porphyromonas spp
- Prevotella spp
- Veillonella spp

*spp - Latin for *Species pluralis.*

Wounds that are colonized or critically colonized can usually be managed effectively with cleansing and antimicrobial dressings as described in Chapter 1. Wounds that show signs of infection require systemic antibiotics, as well as meticulous wound care with topical antimicrobial dressings (especially important for patients with diminished or absent blood flow to the wound area). The non-touch infrared thermometer is an accurate tool for measuring skin temperature,[3] and a study by Maliyar found that measurements on the mirror image of the contralateral leg were significant when combined with two of the other signs and symptoms; however, measurements on the opposite side of the involved leg (e.g. anterior versus posterior) were not significant.[2] Figures 8-1 to 8-6 illustrate wounds with signs and symptoms of both local critical colonization and surrounding infection.

Clinical Guideline: Wounds that have been present less than one month should be treated for gram-positive microbes. If the wound has been present more than one month or if the patient is immune-compromised (e.g. diabetes, HIV, chemotherapy) treatment should be directed toward gram-positive, gram-negative, and anaerobic organisms.[4]

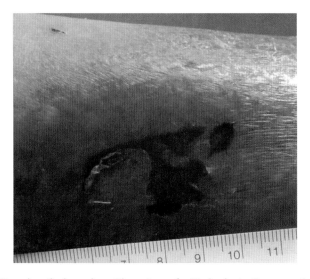

FIGURE 8-1. Wound on the lower leg with no signs of critical colonization; expected to heal with standard care.

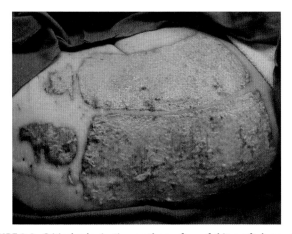

FIGURE 8-2. Critical colonization on the surface of skin graft donor site.

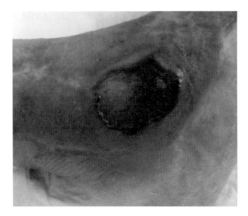

FIGURE 8-3. Critical colonization suspected on the lateral malleolus wound that has friable granulation tissue.

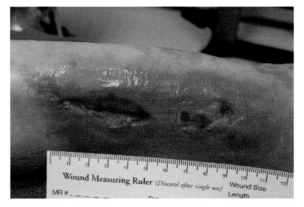

FIGURE 8-4. Wound infection as noted by erythema of periwound tissue.

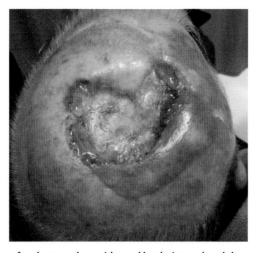

FIGURE 8-5. Infection of scalp wound as evidenced by drainage, breakdown of new epithelium, and erythema of periwound tissue.

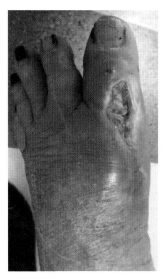

FIGURE 8-6. Forefoot infection and dehisced incision as a result of infected hardware after bunionectomy.

CELLULITIS

Figures 8-7 through 8-17

Pathophysiology

- An acute bacterial infection of the dermis and subcutaneous tissue caused most frequently by *streptococci* or *staphylococci*
- Entry of bacteria can be through a break in the skin, except in the face where skin injury is usually not observed
- Includes the following risk factors: venous edema, lymphedema, pre-existing skin conditions, traumatic injury, leg wounds, peripheral vascular disease, fungal infections, past history of cellulitis, obesity[5,6]

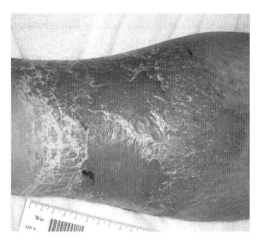

FIGURE 8-7. Cellulitis on the lower leg (note irregular border at proximal edge).

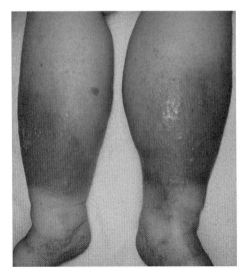

FIGURE 8-8. Bilateral lower extremity cellulitis associated with lymphedema.

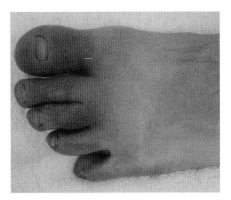

FIGURE 8-9. Cellulitis in first and third toes.

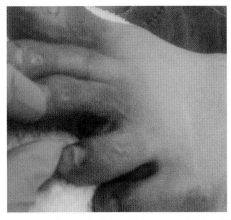

FIGURE 8-10. Portal of entry for bacteria between third and fourth toes.

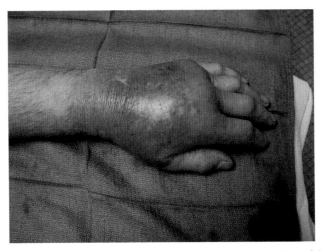

FIGURE 8-11. Cellulitis of the hand; portal of entry is a small wound at the base of the thumb.

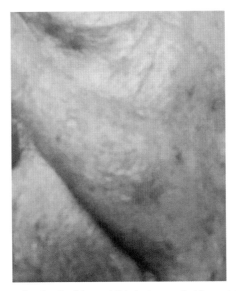

FIGURE 8-12. Cellulitis on the cheek with no visible lesion; probable portal for bacteria is the oral cavity, e.g. gums.

> **Diagnostic Clue:** Erysipelas is a superficial bacterial infection of the upper dermis and subcutaneous lymphatic vessels which can be differentiated from cellulitis by its well-demarcated, more raised appearance. It causes the skin to be bright red, inflamed, and rough.

Clinical presentation
- Presents with local signs (pain, erythema, warmth, and edema) and systemic signs (fever, chills, tachycardia, and leukocytosis)[7,8] (Table 8-3)
- Has uneven erythematous borders; may or may not blanche with pressure
- Occurs ≈ 60% in the lower extremities; other locations include face, arms, hands, and feet[9]

TABLE 8-3.   ALT-70 cellulitis score

The following scoring system, based on clinical symptoms, was developed to help differentiate pseudo-cellulitis (score 0–2 points) from acute cellulitis (score ≥5 points):

Asymmetry—3 points

Leukocytosis—1 point

Tachycardia—1 point

Age ≥70 years—2 points

Data from Raff AB, Weng QY, Cohen JM, et al. A predictive model for diagnosis of lower extremity cellulitis: A cross-sectional study, J Am Acad Dermatol 2017 Apr;76(4):618-625.

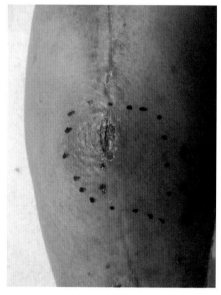

FIGURE 8-13. Erythema is marked with an indelible pen to monitor progression or regression.

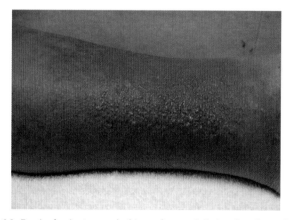

FIGURE 8-14. Erysipelas (note rough skin surface and distinct border at distal edge).

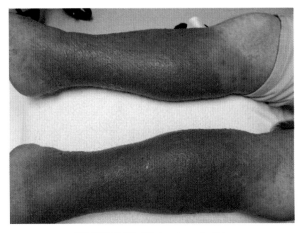

FIGURE 8-15. Bilateral erysipelas.

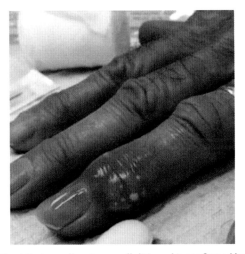

FIGURE 8-16. Gout that can disguise as cellulitis and is confirmed by tissue culture.

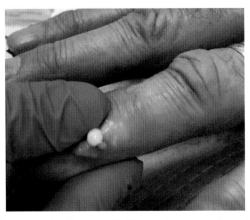

FIGURE 8-17. Clinically, the exudate from gout is fibrous whereas purulence is more homogeneous.

Medical management
- Tests to rule out other potential causes of similar signs and symptoms (e.g. deep vein thrombosis, deeper abscess, necrotizing fasciitis)
- Oral antibiotics,[10] with 12 days of treatment suggested to have fewer cases of recurrence[11]
- Surgical debridement of any necrotic tissue or existing abscesses

Wound management
- Antimicrobial dressings to any open areas, covered with absorbent dressings for drainage
- Compression of the lower extremity, based on vascular status, to eliminate edema that often accompanies cellulitis
- Lymphedema compression contra-indicated until cellulitis is effectively treated[12]

NECROTIZING FASCIITIS (NF)

Figures 8-18 through 8-20

Pathophysiology
- A rapidly-progressing bacterial infection of the soft tissue which travels along the fascial plane, resulting in necrosis of the subcutaneous tissue, fascia, and muscles
- Two classifications of NF include:
  - Type 1: polymicrobial involving at least one anaerobe with or without a facultative anaerobe; localizes on the trunk, abdomen, or perineum
  - Type 2: monomicrobial caused mainly by group A beta hemolytic streptococci and/or other streptococci or staphylococci; occurs mainly on the extremities[13]
- Most common risk factor is diabetes (possibly causing an increase in the number of pediatric cases); followed by immune suppression, renal failure, liver cirrhosis, pulmonary diseases, malignancy, obesity, malnutrition, and last injection drug abuse[13]
- Frequently occurs after a minor skin trauma or surgical procedure that becomes a portal for the bacteria, especially in children[14]
- Bacteria release toxins that produce an exotoxin that in turn activates T cells. This process produces increased cytokines that in turn leads to toxic shock syndrome.

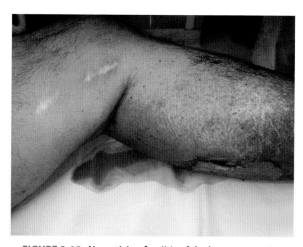

FIGURE 8-18. Necrotizing fasciitis of the lower extremity.

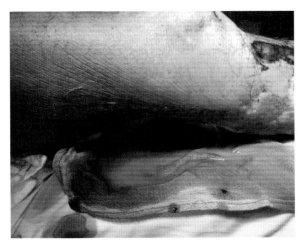

FIGURE 8-19. "Dishwater" drainage, induration, and open wounds typical of necrotizing fasciitis.

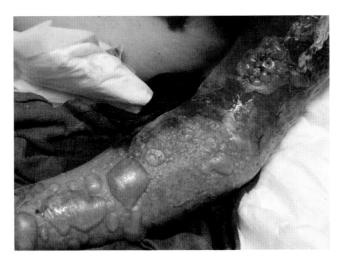

FIGURE 8-20. Necrotizing fasciitis of the upper extremity that developed after shoulder surgery.

> **Diagnostic Clue:** NF in the perineal and genital areas is diagnosed as Fournier's gangrene. Risk factors include penetrating trauma, recent surgery, and immunosuppressed conditions such as diabetes and neutropenia. Fournier's gangrene occurs most frequently in males, age over 50 years, and with history of alcohol abuse.[15] Treatment is essentially the same as for NF.

Clinical presentation
- Early local signs include edema, induration, and erythema and is thus often misdiagnosed as cellulitis
- Early systemic signs include fever, severe pain (out of proportion to the clinical findings), tachycardia, elevated white blood count[14]
- Lack of adenopathy; bacteria miss immune recognition

- Late local signs include blistering and skin necrosis, hypothesia, or anesthesia
- Gray or "dishwater" colored drainage from the wound[16]
- Striking indifference to one's clinical state
- Toxic shock appearance with rapid demise
- The LRINEC scoring tool assesses probability of NF diagnosis in the emergency room (Table 8-4)
- Low serum procalcitonin (<0.87 ng/ml) has also been associated with a high probability of having NF[17]

Medical management
- Immediate initiation of broad-spectrum IV antibiotics
- *Emergent* surgical debridement of all infected tissue; may require subsequent surgical debridement as well as on-going sharp debridement of necrotic tissue with dressing changes
- Medical stabilization as needed
- Plastic reconstruction as soon as wounds are clean and granulated

Wound management
- Antimicrobial dressings (nanocrystalline silver, half or quarter strength Dakin's if there is no granulation tissue present, cadexomer iodine)
- Serial debridement of any necrotic tissue with every dressing change
- Negative pressure wound therapy with antibiotic instillation
- Rehab services to maintain range of motion, preserve strength, and optimize function

TABLE 8-4.   The LRINEC (Laboratory Risk Indicator for Necrotizing Fasciitis) score to differentiate necrotizing fasciitis from cellulitis

C Reactive Protein (mg/L)	<150	0
	≥150	4
White Blood Cell (cells/mm³)	<15	0
	15–25	1
	>25	2
Hemoglobin (g/dL)	>13.5	0
	11.1–13.5	1
	<11	2
Sodium (mmol/L)	>135	0
	<135	2
Creatinine (mg/dL)	<1.6	0
	>1.6	2
Glucose (mg/dL)	<180	0
	>180	1

Interpretation: 0–5, less than 50% probability for developing NF; 6–7, 50–75% risk of having NF; >8, more than 75% risk of having NF. Score has high specificity but low sensitivity.
Reproduced with permission from Wong CH, Khin LW, Heng KS, et al: The LRINEC (Laboratory Risk Indicator for Necrotizing Fasciitis) score: a tool for distinguishing necrotizing fasciitis from other soft tissue infections, Crit Care Med 2004 Jul;32(7):1535-1541.

OSTEOMYELITIS

Figures 8-21 through 8-26

Pathophysiology

- Is infection of the bone with the following three stages:
  - Stage 1: the pathogen, usually *Staphylococcus aureus,* invades the medullary canal of the involved bone and becomes a nidus of infection
  - Stage 2: the acute phase during which the infection results in purulence which spreads to the vascular channels in the bone
  - Stage 3: the chronic phase, a result of the inflammatory processes obliterating the vascular channels with subsequent ischemia and bone necrosis[18]
- Is classified as hematogenous or exogenous
  - Hematogenous: caused by pathogens carried in the bloodstream from sites of infection in other parts of the body
  - Exogenous: caused by pathogens that enter from outside the body (e.g. open fractures, surgical sites, penetrating wounds)[19]

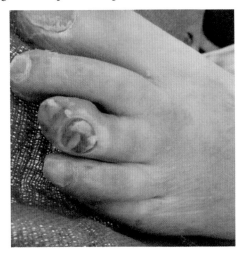

FIGURE 8-21. Osteomyelitis of the third toe, with exposed bone.

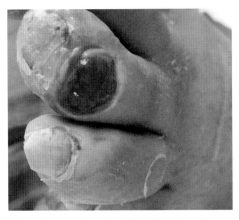

FIGURE 8-22. Two weeks later, the same toe after IV antibiotics and removal of the necrotic bone.

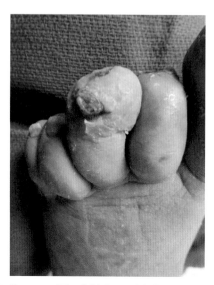

FIGURE 8-23. Osteomyelitis of third toe with the "sausage" appearance.

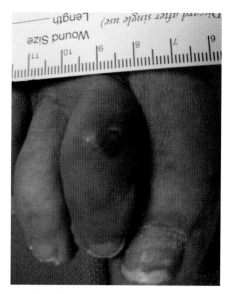

FIGURE 8-24. Osteomyelitis of third toe with erythema and the "sausage" appearance.

Clinical presentation
- Acute hematogenous osteomyelitis
  - Occurs usually in children, especially with sickle cell disease
  - Affects the long bones (femur, tibia, humerus, pelvis)
  - Presents with focal tenderness, swelling, difficulty with weight-bearing activities[9]

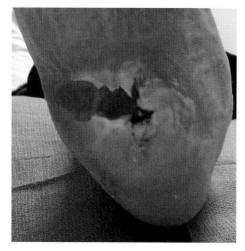

FIGURE 8-25. Osteomyelitis of calcaneus, suspected and confirmed by probing with metal forceps to palpate exposed bone.

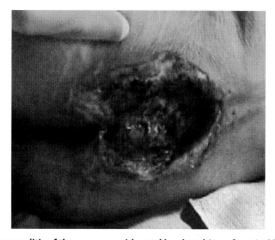

FIGURE 8-26. Osteomyelitis of the sacrum, evidenced by sloughing of cortical layer of bone due to the inflammatory response in trabecular bone.

- Chronic osteomyelitis
  - Occurs usually in adults; usually occurs in the small bones of the foot if the patient has diabetes
  - Presents with symptoms about 1 month after the introduction of a pathogen
  - Presents with low-grade fever, drainage, pain, loss of bone stability; in patients with diabetes, may present with elevated glucose levels
  - Causes over-lying soft tissue infection with edema, erythema, and possible necrosis
  - May cause exposed bone in the wound bed of patients with diabetes[20,21]

> **Diagnostic Clue:** If a patient with diabetes has elevated glucose levels and an adequate hemoglobin A1c, the infection is causing elevated glucose levels and treatment will address the infection; diabetes medications stay the same. However, if the hemoglobin A1c is high, the blood glucose has been uncontrolled for several months, and treatment needs to address both the blood sugars (i.e. change diabetes medication) and the infection.[22]

Medical management
- Diagnosis
  - Identification of the pathogen through bone biopsy (gold standard for diagnosis)
- Treatment
  - Surgical debridement for wounds that include tissue invasion, abscess, open purulence, fistulae, or acute osteomyelitis (all of which can lead to sepsis)
  - Pathogen-specific antibiotics for at least 6 weeks, usually by IV

Wound management
- Sharp debridement of necrotic and/or infected soft tissue
- Antimicrobial dressings using a delivery material sufficient to manage the amount of wound drainage (e.g. foam, alginate, cellulose, or cadexomer iodine paste)
- Ultraviolet C for bacterial reduction
- Removable off-loading footwear in the case of plantar diabetic foot ulcers (total contact cast contra-indicated until infection is resolved)
- Negative pressure wound therapy with instillation of antimicrobial solution on larger wounds or after surgical debridement

HERPES VIRAL INFECTIONS

Figures 8-27 **through** 8-32
- Varicella virus that presents in three ways
  - Herpes simplex type 1 (oral or cold sores)
  - Herpes simplex type 2 (genital herpes)
  - Herpes zoster (chicken pox and shingles)
- Herpes simplex virus
  - Is a DNA virus that invades the muco-epithelial cell nucleus and replicates, thereby producing partial thickness wounds
  - Causes the following pathological changes: multinucleated giant cells, degeneration of epithelial cells, focal necrosis, eosinophilic intra-nuclear inclusion bodies, and an inflammatory response[23]
  - Travels retrograde to the sensory neurons (trigeminal ganglion in type 1 and dorsal root or sacral ganglion in type 2)[23]
  - Persists in the individual for a lifetime due to the presence of a latent pool of the virus in terminally differentiated neurons, usually the peripheral ganglion,[24] and is reactivated by the following precipitating factors: exposure to ultraviolet light, sunlight, fever, excitement, emotional stress, or trauma (e.g. oral intubation)[23]
  - Has multiple lesions (mean is 20), is bilateral and extensive (herpes simplex type 2)[23]
  - Can cause complications in immune-suppressed individuals, e.g. chronic herpetic ulcers, local and systemic infection, and mucous membrane damage[25]

- Herpes zoster virus
  - Is a double-stranded DNA virus that appears at first infection as chicken pox
  - Enters through the respiratory system and infects the tonsillar T cells which carry the virus to the reticuloendothelial system where the major replication occurs, and to the skin where the rash appears (chicken pox)
  - Establishes life-long latency in sensory and autonomic neurons
  - Host develops immunity, but as immunity wanes, latent virus may reactivate years or decades later as herpes zoster (commonly referred to as shingles), usually during a period of stress or immunosuppression[26]
  - Is highly contagious by both contact and airborne transmission

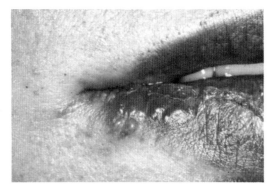

FIGURE 8-27. Initial signs of herpes simplex type 1.

Reproduced with permission from Ryan K, Ahmad N, Alspaugh JA, et al: Sherris Medical Microbiology, 7th ed. New York, NY: McGraw Hill; 2018.

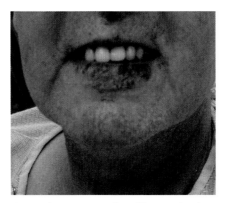

FIGURE 8-28. Later progression of herpes simplex type 1.

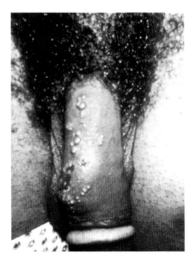

FIGURE 8-29. Herpes simplex type 2.

Reproduced with permission from Ryan K, Ahmad N, Alspaugh JA, et al: Sherris Medical Microbiology, 7th ed. New York, NY: McGraw Hill; 2018.

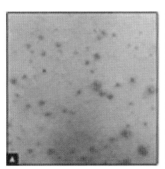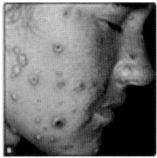

FIGURE 8-30. Herpes zoster (chicken pox).

Reproduced with permission from Goldsmith LA, Katz SI, Gilchrest BA et al: Fitzpatrick's Dermatology in General Medicine, 8th ed. New York, NY: McGraw Hill; 2012.

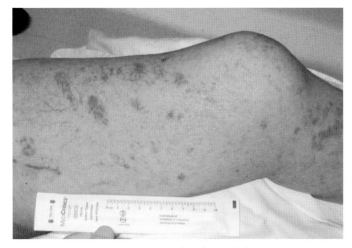

FIGURE 8-31. Herpes zoster (shingles), initial presentation.

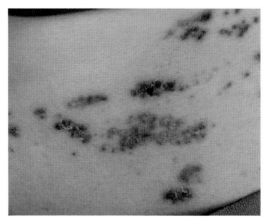

FIGURE 8-32. Herpes zoster (shingles), later presentation.

Clinical presentation
- Herpes simplex type 1
  - Occurs on the lips and mouth
  - Usually occurs initially during childhood, tends to be recurrent
  - Progresses through the stages of prodrome, erythema, papule, vesicle, ulcer, hard crust, and residual dry flaking and swelling
  - Lasts from 3 days (non-ulcerative lesions) to 7–10 days (ulcerative lesions)
  - Can spread to eyes (herpes keratitis) with complaints of eye pain, discharge, and a gritty feeling beneath the eye lid
- Herpes simplex type 2
  - Watery blisters in the genital area
  - Pain during urination
  - Pruritis
  - May also exhibit systemic signs of fever, swollen lymph nodes, headaches, fatigue, or decreased appetite
- Chicken pox
  - Fever and malaise
  - Pruritic rash that starts on the face, scalp, and trunk; spreads to the extremities
  - Begins as maculopapules and rapidly progresses to vesicles, then pustules that rupture, and then to crusts
- Shingles
  - Grouped vesicles on an erythematous base limited to a single dermatome
  - May begin with pain, burning sensation, or tingling in the affected dermatome 48–72 hours before the onset of lesions, which may appear 3–5 days later
  - Become vesicles, then rupture, ulcerate, and crust
  - Usually resolves in 10–15 days
  - May cause post-herpatic neuralgia of varying severity
  - Tends to be more severe and longer lasting in immune-compromised individuals[27]

Medical management
- Herpes simplex type 1
  - Prescription anti-viral creams (Acyclovir and Penciclovir)
- Herpes simplex type 2
  - Antiviral medication (Acyclovir, Famciclovir, Valcyclovir)
  - Education on strategies necessary to prevent transmission to others
- Chicken pox
  - Usually heals in less than 2 weeks with no intervention
  - Varicella vaccine at 12 months or older if there are no contraindications
- Shingles
  - Antiviral medication, to be administered as soon as possible after diagnosis
  - Airborne precautions if patient is hospitalized for any reason
  - Prophylactic vaccine (Shingrix) for adults over 50 years of age,[27] administered twice, 2–6 months apart

Wound management
- Herpes simplex type 1
  - Anti-viral creams (Docosanol)
- Herpes simplex type 2
  - Topical acyclovir
  - Mild corticosteroid ointment for itching
- Chicken pox
  - No wound care indicated
- Shingles
  - Moisture retentive dressings such as hydrogels, hydrocolloids, transparent films, or alginates to facilitate autolytic debridement and healing, as well as to protect the lesions from friction and pressure[28]

TINEA INFECTIONS

Figures 8-33 **through** 8-45

Pathophysiology
- Tinea (the Latin word for "worm") are specific fungal infections that occur in areas that contain keratin (e.g. hair, nails, stratum corneum)
- The fungi penetrate the stratum corneum, invade the keratin, and produce the enzyme keratinase which enables the fungi to use keratin as a source of nutrition
- Primary species are Trichophyton, Microsporum, and Epidermophyton
- May also be caused by non-dermatophyte molds or yeasts (e.g. *candida*)[29]
- Patients at risk for tinea infections include the following:
  - Those who live in crowded and humid conditions
  - Those who perspire excessively in areas where the fungi can thrive (arm pits, groin, abdominal folds)
  - Those who participate in contact sports
  - Those who wear tight constrictive clothing
  - Those with compromised immune systems[30]

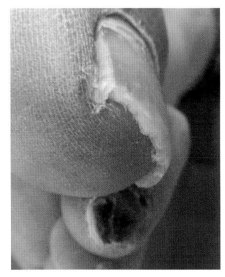

FIGURE 8-33. Onychomycosis with the "cottage cheese" appearance under the nail.

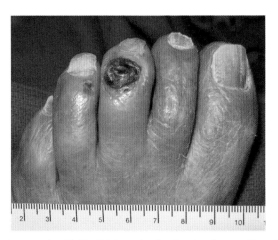

FIGURE 8-34. Onychomycosis with the thickened nails, discoloration, and banding of the great toe nail.

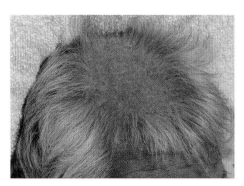

FIGURE 8-35. Tinea capitis.

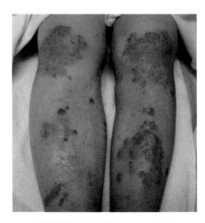

FIGURE 8-36. Tinea corporis.

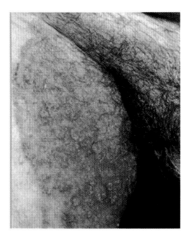

FIGURE 8-37. Tinea cruris.
Reproduced with permission from Kang S, Amagai M, Bruckner AL, et al: Fitzpatrick's Dermatology, 9th ed. New York, NY: McGraw Hill; 2019.

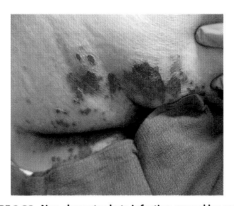

FIGURE 8-38. Non-dermatophyte infection caused by *candida.*

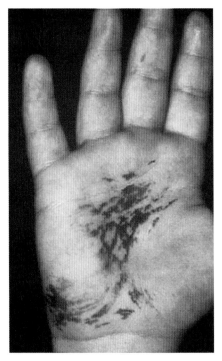

FIGURE 8-39. Tinea nigra.
Reproduced with permission from Kang S, Amagai M, Bruckner AL, et al: Fitzpatrick's Dermatology, 9th ed. New York, NY: McGraw Hill; 2019.

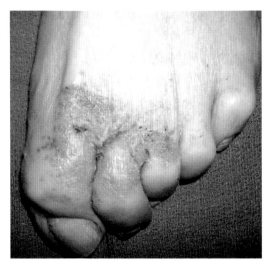

FIGURE 8-40. Tinea pedis.

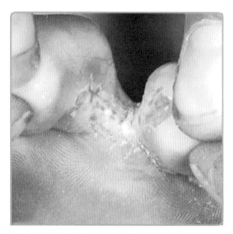

FIGURE 8-41. Tinea pedis with maceration between the toes.
Reproduced with permission from Kang S, Amagai M, Bruckner AL, et al: Fitzpatrick's Dermatology, 9th ed. New York, NY: McGraw Hill; 2019.

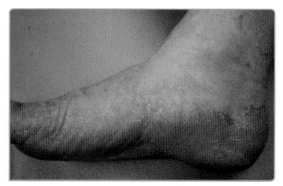

FIGURE 8-42. Tinea pedis with scaling and peeling.
Reproduced with permission from Kang S, Amagai M, Bruckner AL, et al: Fitzpatrick's Dermatology, 9th ed. New York, NY: McGraw Hill; 2019.

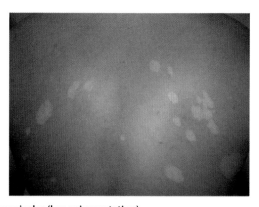

FIGURE 8-43. Tinea versicolor (hypopigmentation).
Reproduced with permission from Usatine RP, Smith MA, Mayeaux EJ, et al: The Color Atlas and Synopsis of Family Medicine, 3rd ed. New York, NY: McGraw Hill; 2019. Photo contributor: Richard P. Usatine, MD.

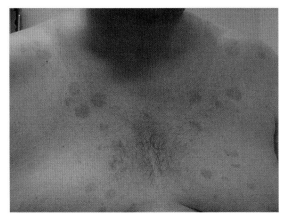

FIGURE 8-44. Tinea versicolor (hyperpigmentation).

Reproduced with permission from Usatine RP, Smith MA, Mayeaux EJ, et al: The Color Atlas and Synopsis of Family Medicine, 3rd ed. New York, NY: McGraw Hill; 2019. Photo contributor: Richard P. Usatine, MD.

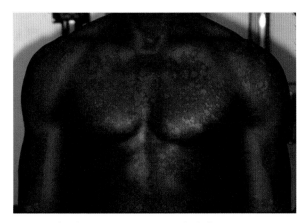

FIGURE 8-45. Tinea versicolor (hypopigmentation) on dark skin.

Reproduced with permission from Usatine RP. What is in a name? West J Med 2000 Oct;173(4):231-232.

Clinical presentation
- Tinea infections are named according to the body part affected; clinical signs can differ depending on the area. Names and clinical signs are presented in Table 8-5.

Medical management
- Topical and systemic antifungal medications depending on the area affected and the severity of the disease. See Table 8-5.

Clinical Guidelines: A clinical pathway developed by Gupta, et al., recommends the following guidelines for treating onychomycosis, based on the amount of nail involvement: terbinafine for severe (>60% involvement); terbinafine or efinaconazole for moderate (20–60% involvement); efinaconazole for mild (<20% involvement). Co-morbidities, patient preference and adherence, and nail thickness may require the use of alternative oral or topical antifungals.

TABLE 8-5. Name, location, clinical signs, and treatment of tinea infections

Name	Location	Signs & Symptoms	Treatment
Onychomycosis (also called tinea unguium)	Nail plates, especially in individuals who are elderly, immunocompromised, or have diabetes or PAD.	• Nail dystrophy • Nail discoloration • Separation of nail from underlying skin • With or without odor • Possible tendency to affect adjacent skin • Possible infection[6]	• Oral antifungal agents Terbinafine Itraconazole (pulse regimen)[1] • Topical fungal agents Efinaconazole Tavaborole[2] • CO_2 laser therapy[3,4] • Urea (in conjunction with topical or oral antifungal treatment)[5]
Tinea capitis	Scalp, usually in pre-puberty children, males more than females Termed tinea barbae when in the beard	• Itching scalp • Patches of hair loss with "black dots" where the hair breaks off • Perifollicular scales and pustules • Trichoscopic findings: Comma or cork-screw hair, Morse code-like hairs, zigzag or bent hairs[6] • May develop kerions, or painful spongy masses with pustules and crusts	• Oral antifungal agents Itraconazole Terbinafine Griseofulvin[6,7]
Tinea corporis (ringworm)	Skin, usually the arms and legs, especially glabrous skin If on the hands, termed tinea manuum	• Enlarged raised red rings with clear centers • Itching • Scales • Hair loss	• Topical azoles • Topical steroid and antifungal combination • Terbinafine • Naftifine[8]
Tinea cruris (jock itch)	Groin, inner thighs, genitals, buttocks	• Itching • Small erythematous, scaling patches • Vesicles with well-defined borders	• Topical azoles • Topical steroid and antifungal combination • Terbinafine • Naftifine[3]

Tinea nigra	Palms or soles, primarily in tropical and subtropical regions	• Well-circumscribed brown-black macules	• Potassium hydroxide test to confirm diagnosis and rule out acral lentiginous melanoma • Topical 2% ketoconazole cream twice daily for two weeks[9]
Tinea pedis	Feet, especially in atheletes whose feet becomes sweaty; can spread to the hands	• Usually begins between the toes • Begins as scaly rash • May cause maceration, peeling, and fissuring of toe interspaces • Causes itching, burning, stinging • Is contagious[10]	• Instruction in good pedal hygiene • Topical antifungal sprays or ointments • Oral antifungal medications for severe cases
Tinea versicolor (pityriasis versicolor)	Upper arms, trunk, and neck where the concentration of sebaceous glands is great; occurs mostly in humid weather[11]	• Well-defined round or egg-shaped macules • White, erythematous, or brown pigment[11]	• Fluconazole • Itraconazole • Pramiconazole[12] • Ketoconazole 2% shampoo[13]

[1]Kreijkamp-Kaspers S, Hawke K, Guo L, Kerin G, Bell-Syer SE, Magin P et al. Oral antifungal medication for toenail onychomycosis. Cochrane Database Syst Rev. 2017 Jul 14;7:CD010031.

[2]Thomas J, Peterson GM, Christenson JK, Kosari S, Baby KE. Antifungal drug use for onychomycosis. Am J Ther. 2019;26(3):e388-e396.

[3]Ma W, Si C, Kasyanju LM, Liu HF, Yin XF, Liu J, et al. Laser treatment for onychomycosis: A systematic review and meta-analysis. Medicine (Baltimore).2019;98(48):e17948.

[4]Yeung K, Ortner VK, Martinussen T, Paasch U, Haedersdal M. Efficacy of laser treatment for onychomycotic nails: A systematic review and meta-analysis of prospective clinical trials. Lasers Med Sci. 2019;34(8):1513-1525.

[5]Dars S, Banwell HA, Matricciani L. The use of urea for the treatment of onychomycosis: A systematic review. J Foot Ankle Res. 2019;Apr 11;12:22. Available at https://doi:10.1186/s13047-019-0332-3. eCollection 2019. Accessed April 18, 2020.

[6]Waskiel-Burnat A, Rakowska A, Sikora M, Ciechanowicz P, Olszewska M, Rudnicka L. Trichoscopy of tinea capitis: A systematic review. Dermatol Ther (Heidelb). 2020;10(1):43-52.

[7]Gupta AD, Mays RR, Versteeg SG, Piraccini BM, Shear NH, Piguet V, et al. Tinea capitis in children: A systematic review of management. J Eur Acad Dermatol Venereol. 2018;32(12):2264-2274.

[8]El-Gohary M, vanZuuren EJ, Fedorowicz Z, Burgess H, Doney L, Stuart B, et al. Topical antifungal treatments for tinea cruris and tinea corporis. Cochrane Database Syst Rev. 2014; Aug 4;(8):CD009992.

[9]Eksomtramage T, Aiempanakit K. Tinea nigra mimicking acral melanocytic nevi. IDCases. 2019;18:e00654. Available at https://doi.org/10.1016/j.dcr.2019.e00654. Accessed April 18, 2020.

[10]Thapa RK, Choi JY, Han SD, Lee GH, Yong CS, Jun J, Kim JO. Therapeutic effects of a novel DA5505 formulation on a guinea pig model of tinea pedis. Dermatologica Sinica. 2017;35:59-65.

[11]El-Housiny S, Eldeen M, El-Attar YA, Salem HA, Atia D, Bendas ER, El-Nabarawi. Fluconazole-loaded solid lipid nanoparticles topical gel for treatment of pityriasis versicolor: Formulation and clinical study. Drug Deliv. 2018;25(1):78-90.

[12]Gupta AK, Lane D, Paquet M. Systematic review of systemic treatments for tinea versicolor an evidence-based dosing regimen recommendation. J Cutan Med Surg. 2014;18(2):79-90.

[13]Lange D, Richards HM, Guarnieri J, Humeniuk JM, Savin RC, Reyes BA, et al. Ketononazole 2% shampoo in the treatment of tinea versicolor: A multicenter, randomized, double-blind, placebo-controlled trial. J Am Acad Dermat. 1998;39(6):944-950.

Wound management
- Educate patient on good hygiene and adherence to treatment
- Use antimicrobial dressings to prevent infection if open lesions appear, usually as a result of scratching

SPOROTRICHOSIS

Figure 8-46

Pathophysiology
- Also called rose gardener's disease; is the most common subcutaneous mycosis
- Caused by the dimorphic fungus *Sporothrix schenckii*[32]
- Has three main forms: lymphocutaneous (most common), fixed cutaneous, and disseminated cutaneous
- Presents at sites of trauma, usually face or extremities
- Occurs with outdoor activity, e.g. gardening, with direct contact with soil, or with contact with domestic cats who carry the fungus on their fur[32]

Clinical presentation
- Initially presents as an erythematous granulomatous nodule at the site of the initial injury, 2–4 mm in diameter, and may ulcerate
- Usually painless
- Spreads proximally via the lymphatics over a course of 1–4 weeks
- If inhaled, can lead to pulmonary infection and subsequently spread to other organs[33]

Medical management
- Systemic antifungal medications, including itraconazole, fluconazole, terbinafine, amphotericin B, or saturated solution of potassium iodide.[28]

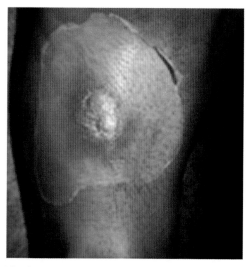

FIGURE 8-46. **Sporotrichosis.**

Reproduced with permission from Knoop KJ, Stack LB, Storrow AB, et al: The Atlas of Emergency Medicine, 4th ed. New York, NY: McGraw Hill; 2016. Photo contributor: Edward J. Otten, MD.

Wound management
- Topical antifungal agents
- Topical application of saturated solution of potassium iodide
- Topical application of heat (the sprorotrichosis organism grows at low temperatures)[28]

ACTINOMYCOSIS

Figure 8-47

Pathophysiology
- Caused by gram-positive, non-spore forming anaerobic bacilli, the most common being *Actinomycosis israelii* which is normally found in the nose, throat, and genital tract[34]
- Can be associated with local tissue damage caused by neoplastic conditions and irradiation
- Usually accompanied by some other bacteria that facilitate its invasion of the tissue[35]

Clinical presentation
- Varies with location, is chronic and difficult to eliminate
- Develops slowly when on the face and neck, with induration and red or cyanotic skin
- Produces yellow particles, similar to sulfur particles, that carry the bacteria, frequently into the adjacent soft tissue and bone
- With pulmonary involvement, presents with fever, cough, sputum production, night sweats, weight loss, and pleuritic pain[34]

Medical management
- Surgical excision of the infected tissue, followed by plastic reconstruction
- IV or oral antibiotics (beta-lactams such as ampicillin, penicillin, or amoxicillin) for at least 6 months
- Doxycycline or sulfonamides as alternative medications[36]

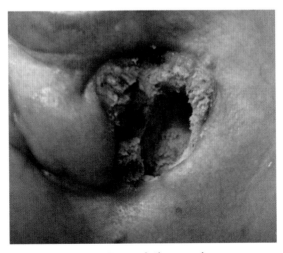

FIGURE 8-47. Actinomycosis.

Wound management
- Topical antibiotic solutions
- Secondary dressings, e.g. foams with adhesive borders, in order to minimize the appearance of tissue deformities that can interfere with community activities

MYCOBACTERIA

Figure 8-48

Pathophysiology
- Typical or atypical mycobacteria (tuberculosis) that are neither gram-positive nor gram-negative may cause skin lesions. (Table 8-6)
- Bacteria replicate intra-cellularly and may become dormant in the host tissue.[37]
- Cutaneous infections usually result from exogenous inoculations.
- Predisposing factors include a history of preceding trauma, immunosuppression, or chronic disease (e.g. diabetes)[28]

Clinical presentation
- Lesions appear 2–4 weeks after inoculation, usually on the hands, lower extremities, or face.
- Lesions are shallow and granular, or have a hemorrhagic base with surrounding abscesses.[37]
- Edges may be ragged with undermining and reddish-blue in color, may become edematous and indurated.
- Lymphadenopathy may develop 3–8 weeks after infection begins.

Medical management
- Diagnosis is made by bacteria culture.
- Primary treatment is chemotherapy with Isoniazid, Rifampicin, Rifapentine, Ethambutol, or Pyrazinamide, or streptomycin.[37]

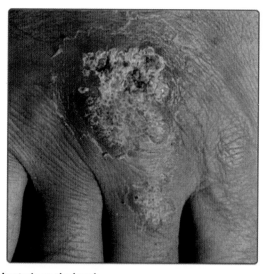

FIGURE 8-48. Mycobacteria on the hand.

Reproduced with permission from Kang S, Amagai M, Bruckner AL, et al: Fitzpatrick's Dermatology, 9th ed. New York, NY: McGraw Hill; 2019.

TABLE 8-6. Mycobacterium species that cause integumentary disorders

Species	Clinical Presentation	Treatment
Mycobacteria tuberculosis species	Abscess	Surgery
Scrofuloderma	Lymphadenopathy	Anti-tuberculous drugs
Lupus vulgaris	Fistulae	
Military lesions	Ulcerations	
Nontuberculous mycobacteria		
M. Marinum	Swimming pool and fish tank granuloma	Anti-tuberculous drugs
M. Ulcerans (Buruli ulcer)	Subcutaneous nodule	Surgical excision
Mavium intracellulare	Small ulcers with erythematous borders	Surgical excision and chemotherapy
M. Kansasii	Crusted ulcerations	Anti-tuberculous drugs, Minocycline,
M. Chelonae	Painful nodules, abscesses, surgical wound infection	Erythromycin, Tobramycin, Amikacin, Doxycycline
M. Fortuitum	Painful nodules, abscesses, surgical wound infections	Amikacin, Doxycycline, Ciprofloxacin, sulfamethoxazole

Reproduced with permission from Hamm RL: Text and Atlas of Wound Diagnosis and Treatment, 2nd ed. New York, NY: McGraw Hill; 2019.

Wound management
- Antimicrobial dressings with absorbent secondary dressings based on the amount of exudate
- Use of aseptic technique during treatment in order to prevent further infection
- Airborne precautions by all care-givers if the strain is tuberculin[28]

REFERENCES

1. Sibbald G, Woo K, Ayello E. Increased bacterial burden and infection: NERDS and STONES. *Wounds UK.* 2007;3(2):25-46.
2. Maliyar K, Persaud-Jaimangal R, Sibbald RG. Associations among skin surface pH, temperature, and bacterial burden in wounds. *Adv Skin Wound Care.* 2020;33(4):180-185.
3. Sibbald Rg, Mufti A, Armstrong DG. Infrared skin thermometry: An underutilized cost-effective tool for routine wound care practice and patient high-risk diabetic foot self-monitoring. *Adv Skin Wound Care.* 2015;28(1):37-44.
4. Dow G, Browne A, Sibbald RG. Infection in chronic wounds: controversies in diagnosis and treatment. *Ostomy Wound Management.* 1999;45(8):23-40.
5. Kumar M, Ngian V, Yeong C, Keighley C, Nguyen HV, Ong BS. Cellulitis in older people over 75 years – are there differences? *Annals of Medicine and Surgery.* 2020;49:37-40.
6. Quirke M, Ayoub F, McCabe A, Boland F, Smith B, O'Sullivan R, Wakai A. Risk factors for nonpurulent leg cellulitis: A systematic review and meta-analysis. *Br J Dermatol.* 2017;177(2):382-394.

7. Raff AB, Weng QY, Cphen JM, Gunasekera BS, Ikhovat J, Wedak P, et al. A predictive model for diagnosis of lower extremity cellulitis: A cross-sectional study. *J Am Acad Dermatol.* 2017;76(4):618-625.e2.

8. Li DG, Dewan AK, Khosravi H, Joyce C, Mostaghimi A. Athe ALT-70 predictive model outperforms thermal imaging for the diagnosis of lower extremity cellulitis: A prospective evaluation. *J Am Acad Dermatol.* 2018;79(6):1076-1080.e1.

9. Patel M, Lee SI, Akyea RK, Grindlay D, Francis N, Levell NJ, Smart P, et al. A systematic review showing the lack of diagnostic criteria and tolls developed for lower-limb cellulitis. *Br J Dermatol.* 2019;181(6):1156-1165.

10. Brindle R, Williams OM, Barton E, Featherstone P. Assessment of antibiotic treatment of cellulitis and erysipelas: A systematic review and meta-analysis. *JAMA Dermatol.* 2019 Jun 12. doi: 10.1001/jamadermatol.2019.0884. Accessed March 25, 2020.

11. Cranendonk DR, Opmeer BC, van Agtmael MA, Branger J, Brinkman K, Hoepelman AIM, et al. Antibiotic treatment for 6 days versus 12 days in patients with severe cellulitis: A multicenter randomized, couble-blind, placebo-controlled, non-inferiority trial. *Clinical Microbiology and Infection.* 2019. Available at https://doi.org/10.1016/j.cmi.2019.09.019. Accessed March 25, 2020.

12. Perdomo M, Hamm R. Lymphedema. In Hamm R, ed. *Text and Atlas of Wound Diagnosis and Treatment.* 2nd ed. New York, NY: McGraw Hill Education. 2019;145-169.

13. Ali SS, Lateef F. Laboratory risk factors for acute necrotizing fasciitis in the emergency setting. *Journal of Acute Disease.* 2016;5(2):114-116.

14. Pfeifle V. Gros SJ, Holland-Cunz S, Kampfen A. Necrotizing fasciitis in children due to minor lesions. *J Pediatr Surg Case Reports.* 2017;25:52-55.

15. Joury A, Mahendra A, Alshehri M, Downing A. Extensive necrotizing fasciitis from Fournier's gangrene. *Urology Case Reports.* 2019. Available at https://doi.org/10.1016/j.eucr.2019.100943. Accessed April 13, 2020.

16. Guevel LH, Shifrin MM. Necrotizing fasciitis in the adult patient: Implications for nurse practitioners. *J Nurse Practioners.* 2020. Available at https://doi.org/10.1016/j.nurpra.2020.02.008.

17. Novoa-Parra CD, Wadhwani J, Puig-Conca A, et al. Usefulness of a risk scale based on procalcitonin for early discrimination between necrotizing fasciitis and cellulitis of the extremities. *Medicina Clinica (English Edition).* 2019;153(9):347-350.

18. Groll ME, Woods T, Salcido R. Osteomyelitis: A context for wound management. *Adv Skin Wound Care.* 2018;31(6):253-262.

19. Mourad LA, McCance KL. Alterations of musculoskeletal function. In: Huether SE, McCance KL, eds. *Understanding Physiology.* St. Louis, MO:Mosby. 2008;1036-1070.

20. Lavery LA, Armstrong DG, Peters EJ, Lipsky BA. Probe-to-bone test for diagnosing diabetic foot osteomyelitis: reliable or relic? *Diabetes Care.* 2007;30(2):270-274.

21. Senneville E, Lipsky BA, Abbas ZG, Aragon-Sanchez J, Diggle M, Embil JM, et al. Diagnosis of infection in the foot in diabetes: A systematic review. *Diabetes Metab Res Rev.* 2020;36(3): Auppl1:e3281. Doi: 10.1002/dmrr.3281.

22. Scarborough P, McGuire J. Diabetes and the diabetic foot. In Hamm R (Ed). *Text and Atlas of Wound Diagnosis and Treatment,* 2nd ed. New York, NY: McGraw Hill Education. 2019;199-234.

23. Herpesviruses. In: Ryan KJ. ed. *Sherris Medical Microbiology.* 7th ed. New York, NY: McGraw-Hill. http://accessmedicine.mhmedical.com/content.aspx?bookid=2268&sectionid=176083540. Accessed April 21, 2020.

24. Suzich JB, Cliffe AR. Strength in adversity: Understanding the pathways to herpes simplex virus reactivation. *Virology.* 2018;522:81-91.

25. Staidov IN, Neykov NV, Kazandjieva JS, Tsankov KK. Is herpes simplex a systemic disease? *Clin Dermatol.* 2015;33(5):551-555.

26. Harbecke R, Jensen NJ, Depledge DP, Johnson GR, Ashbaugh ME, Schmid DS, et al. Recurrent herpes zoster in the Shingles Prevention Study: Are second episodes caused by the same varicella-zoster virus strain? *Vaccine.* 2020;38:150-157.

27. Lachiewicz AM, Srinivas ML. Varicella-zoster virus post-exposure management and prophylaxis: A review. *Preventive Medicine Reports.* 2019;16. Available at https://doi.org.10.1016/j.pmedr.2019.101016. Accessed April 20, 2020.

28. Hamm R, Shah JB. Atypical Wounds. In Hamm R (Ed). *Text and Atlas of Wound Diagnosis and Treatment.* 2nd ed. New York, NY: McGraw Hill Education. 2019;235-268.

29. Dars S, Banwell HA, Matricciani L. The use of urea for the treatment of onychomycosis: A systematic review. *J Foot Ankle Res.* 2019;Apr 11;12:22. Available at https://doi:10.1186/s13047-019-0332-3. eCollection 2019. Accessed April 18, 2020.

30. Tinea Corporis. Available at https://en.wikipedia.org/wiki/Tinea_corporis. Accessed April 17, 2020.

31. Gupta AK, Sibbald RG, Andriessen A, Belley R, Boroditsky A, Botros M, et al. Toenail onychomycosis – A Canadian approach with a new transungal treatment: Development of a clinical pathway. *J Cutan Med Surg.* 2015;19(5):440-449.

32. Larson KN, Pandey S, Hoover W, Sun NZ. Sporotrichosis in the nail – an unusual location and presentation. *JAAD Case Reports.* 2018;4(1):47-49.

33. Zafren K, Thurman RJ, Jones ID. Chapter 16. Environmental Conditions. In: Knoop KJ, Stack LB, Storrow AB, Thurman RJ, eds. *The Atlas of Emergency Medicine.* 3rd ed. New York: McGraw-Hill. 2010. http://www.accessmedicine.com/content.aspx?aID=6005284. Accessed April 21, 2020.

34. Valour F, Senechal A, Dupieux C, et al. Actinomycosis: Etiology, clinical features, diagnosis, treatment, and management. *Infect Drug Resist.* 2014;7:183-197.

35. Bettesworth J, Gill K, Shah J. Primary actinomycosis of the foot: A case report and literature review. *J Am Coll Clin Wound Spec.* 2009;1(3):95-100.

36. Russo TA. Chapter 163. Actinomycosis. In: Longo DL, Fauci AS, Kasper DL, Hauser SL, Jameson JL, Loscalzo J, eds. *Harrison's Principles of Internal Medicine.* 18th ed. New York: McGraw-Hill. 2012. http://www.accessmedicine.com/content.aspx?aID=9094036. Accessed April 21, 2020.

37. Sethi A. Tuberculosis and Infections with Atypical Mycobacteria. In: Kang S, Amagai M, Bruckner AL, Enk AH, Margolis DJ, McMichael AJ, Orringer JS. eds. *Fitzpatrick's Dermatology.* 9th ed. New York, NY: McGraw-Hill. http://accessmedicine.mhmedical.com/content.aspx?bookid=2570&sectionid=210431641. Accessed April 22, 2020.

9

Malignant Wounds

INTRODUCTION

Most malignant dermal wounds are caused by over-exposure to ultraviolet light or by metastatic spread from a remote neoplasm to the skin; however, some malignancies can cause dermal lesions. In addition some chronic wounds and cutaneous scars, especially from burns, can transition into neoplastic lesions (termed Marjolin's ulcer)[1] and require a totally different plan of care in order to achieve full wound closure. Some of the signs that a wound may be a neoplasm, either benign or malignant, are the following:

- Unusual appearance
- Easy bleeding
- Hypergranulation
- Rapid growth
- Failure to respond to standard care
- Repeated reoccurrence after apparent closure
- Unusual odor
- Pain
- Exudate
- Edema

Along with these physical symptoms come emotional stress, functional compromise, social concerns, and complications such as infection.[2] Any wound that is even suspicious of being malignant requires immediate confirmation or negation by tissue biopsy.

The objective of this chapter is to present the subtle characteristics of malignant wounds and the immediate medical care that is recommended to prevent further metastasis or wound complications. Palliative care for fungating or terminal illness wounds will also be discussed.

BASAL CELL CARCINOMA (BCC)

Figures 9-1 through 9-8

Pathophysiology
- Is the most common skin cancer, and the most frequently occurring cancer overall
- Arises from damaged undifferentiated basal cells

- Is the result of prolonged exposure to ultraviolet (sun or tanning bed) light which leads to the formation of thymine dimers, a form of DNA damage
- Occurs when the DNA damage is greater than what the cells can naturally repair[3]
- Involves the following risk factors:
  - Prolonged ultraviolet exposure in the sun or tanning beds
  - Fair skin, red or blond hair, or light-colored eyes
  - Radiation therapy for other skin conditions
  - Family history of skin cancer
  - Immunosuppression, including anti-rejection medication
  - Exposure to arsenic in water or industry
  - Certain inherited genetic disorders (e.g. Gorlin-Goltz syndrome, xeroderma pigmentosum)[4]

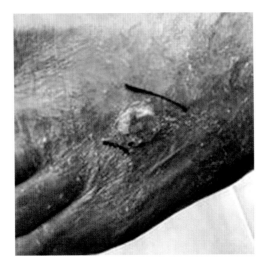

FIGURE 9-1. Basal cell carcinoma (BCC).

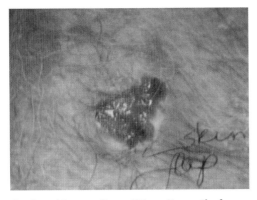

FIGURE 9-2. BCC that developed 7 years after an IV insertion on the forearm.

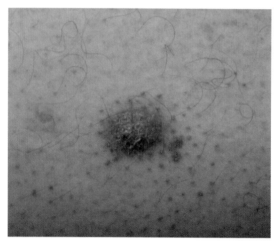

FIGURE 9-3. Early-stage nodular BCC.

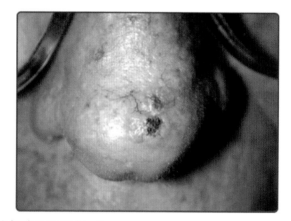

FIGURE 9-4. BCC that has crusted on the nose.
Reproduced with permission from Kang S, Amagai M, Bruckner AL, et al: Fitzpatrick's Dermatology, 9th ed. New York, NY: McGraw Hill; 2019.

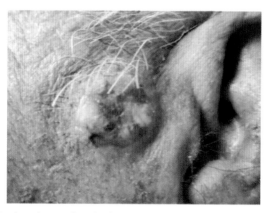

FIGURE 9-5. BCC that has ulcerated on the face.

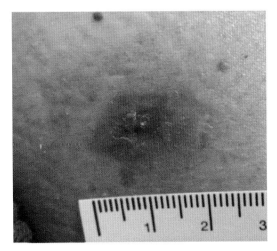

FIGURE 9-6. Infiltrative BCC.

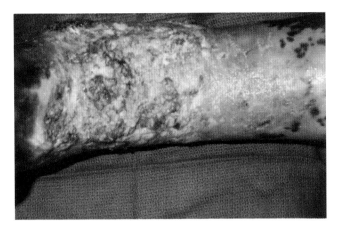

FIGURE 9-7. Ulcerative BCC that was not treated for more than 1½ years, resulting in below-knee amputation.

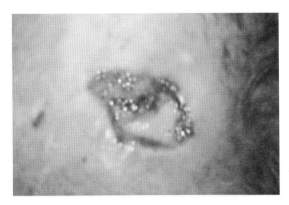

FIGURE 9-8. Excision of a BCC that failed to heal after 6 weeks due to application of hydrogen peroxide twice daily.

Clinical presentation
- Most commonly occurs on the head, face, neck, or extremities where skin is exposed to sun, but can occur anywhere on the body
- Can begin as a small pearly-white, scaly lesion that outgrows its blood supply, erodes, and eventually ulcerates. Can also form as a non-healing or expanding chronic rash.
- May bleed easily with any scraping or friction
- May have prominent telangiectatic surface vessels, rolled edges, or slightly raised dome shape
- Is painless and slow growing[5]
- May develop as a result of a non-healing traumatic wound[1]
- Presents as three types:
  - Nodular—appears as shiny, pearly skin
  - Superficial—appears as a red patch, may be mistaken for eczema
  - Infiltrative—(also called morpheaform) appears as thickened skin or scar tissue; penetrates deeper and is harder to treat; is more aggressive[6]

Medical management
- Biopsy of any suspicious lesion with anesthetic and surgical shaving technique. It is essential that the biopsy is not too shallow and obtains a depth to the dermis.
- Surgical excision or Mohs procedure until there are 4 mm (excision) or 2 mm (Mohs) clean margins
- Cryosurgery (Sufficient enough to treat the lesion as well as have a margin of normal skin and acceptable depth)
- Electrodessication and curettage (Sufficient enough to treat the lesion as well as have a margin of normal skin and acceptable depth)
- Topical 5% imiquimod cream daily, 6 weeks for superficial BCC or 12 weeks for nodular BCC[7]; 5-Fluorourcil[8]; or vismodegib[9]
- Radiotherapy for elder patients or for areas where excision would be disfiguring
- Photodynamic therapy for primary superficial BCCs only
- Recommendation of avoiding sun and tanning beds and of using at least 30 SPF sunscreen
- Follow-up full-body skin inspection by a dermatologist to detect recurrence or new lesions

Wound management
- Avoid cytotoxic agents (e.g. hydrogen peroxide, Dakin's solution, acetic acid) after any excision procedures. (Figure 9-8)
- Treat any open areas after excision with moist wound therapy.

SQUAMOUS CELL CARCINOMA (SCC)

*Figures 9-9 **through** 9-16*

Pathophysiology
- Is a malignant neoplasm of the keratinizing epidermal cells with histological evidence of full epidermal involvement (superficial SCC) or invasion to the dermis or deeper tissue (invasive SCC)
- Has DNA mutations that prevent normal squamous cell apoptosis, resulting in uncontrolled over-growth of the cells

- Is termed a Marjolin's ulcer if the SCC occurs in the area of a previous wound (e.g. burn, trauma, venous ulcer, osteomyelitis, etc.) and is usually very aggressive[10,11,12]
  - May have a latency period
  - Occurs most frequently in burn scar sites, or scars and non-healing wounds that have repeated irritation, friction, or other mechanical stress on the tissue
  - Has a male-to-female ratio of 2:1[12]
- Associated with the following risk factors:
  - Exposure to ultraviolet A and B light, or ionizing radiation
  - Exposure to toxins such as arsenic
  - Fair skin and blue eyes
  - History of radiation therapy
  - Anti-rejection medication after organ transplant (Figure 9-15)

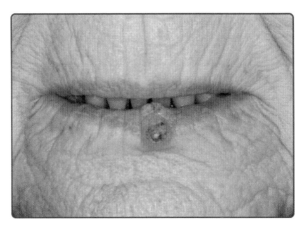

FIGURE 9-9. SCC on the lip.
Reproduced with permission from Kang S, Amagai M, Bruckner AL, et al: Fitzpatrick's Dermatology, 9th ed. New York, NY: McGraw Hill; 2019.

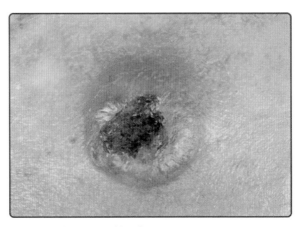

FIGURE 9-10. SCC with raised periwound border.
Reproduced with permission from Kang S, Amagai M, Bruckner AL, et al: Fitzpatrick's Dermatology, 9th ed. New York, NY: McGraw Hill; 2019.

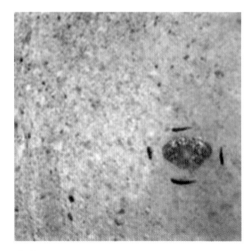

FIGURE 9-11. SCC (invasive).

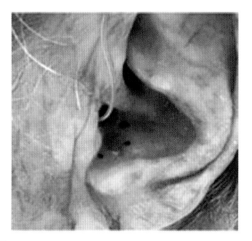

FIGURE 9-12. SCC in the ear.

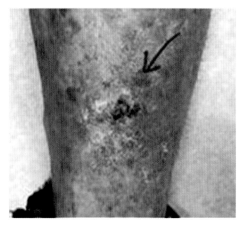

FIGURE 9-13. SCC with scaly surrounding skin.

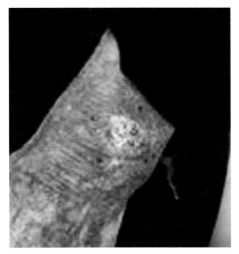

FIGURE 9-14. SCC with a scaly crust.

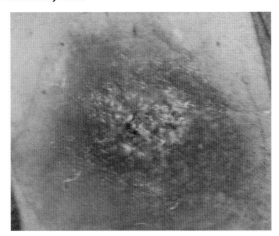

FIGURE 9-15. SCC on a patient who had double lung transplant with subsequent anti-rejection medication.

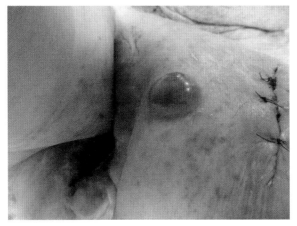

FIGURE 9-16. New dermal SCC lesion that occurred after radiation for metastatic SCC disease.

Clinical presentation
- Can present as a firm smooth red papule, nodule, or plaque (invasive SCC)
- Can present as a non-healing or expanding scaly chronic rash (superficial SCC)
- May progress to a lesion with a scaly crust
- May have poorly defined edges and a scaly surrounding skin
- Is commonly hyperkeratotic or ulcerated
- May sometimes metastasize rapidly

> **Diagnostic Clue:** When the lesion is a cutaneous eruption from a deeper malignancy, SCC often appears first as a nodule that subsequently ulcerates. This may be a sign of recurring metastasis with a poor prognosiss (Figure 9-16).

Medical management
- Sufficiently deep-shave biopsy to confirm diagnosis
- Surgical excision, electrodessication and curettage, or cryotherapy for smaller SCCs[5]
- Mohs micrographic surgery (highest cure rate overall) for larger, higher risk SCCs, or SCCs located on higher risk areas (head/hands/feet/genitals)[13]

Wound management
- Standard, supportive wound care for radiated tissue and open wounds that may occur as a result of treatment (See Chapter 6 on Burns for more information on treating radiation wounds.)
- Antimicrobial dressings and septic technique to prevent infection
- Non-adherent, absorbent dressings to manage pain and exudate
- Lymphedema management
- Frequent skin inspections for any new lesions, an indication that any underlying malignancy may be recurring

MELANOMA

Figures 9-17 through 9-22

Pathophysiology
- Is an aggressive skin cancer that involves the melanocytes in the basal layer of the epidermis
- Is abnormal growth of melanocytes that are unable to respond appropriately to regulatory cues from keratinocytes as a result of mutation in the genes that regulate cell growth
- May originate as a nevus or mole which is formed when there is an overlap in the growth involving both the epidermis and dermis[14]
- May also originate from transformed stem cells, in which case the melanoma may be resistant to treatment[15]
- Can occur as new, abnormally appearing moles or freckles
- Occurs most frequently in areas that are exposed to ultraviolet light from the sun or from tanning beds, but can occur in the eyes, nails, genitals, and non-sun exposed areas
- Presents in the following types:
  - Superficial spreading malignant melanoma

- ○ Nodular melanoma
- ○ Acral lentiginous melanoma
- ○ Minimal deviation melanoma
- ○ Desmoplastic melanoma
- ○ Amelanotic melanoma (lacks typical pigmentation of most melanomas, and can mimic SCC, BCC, or other nodular red cancers)

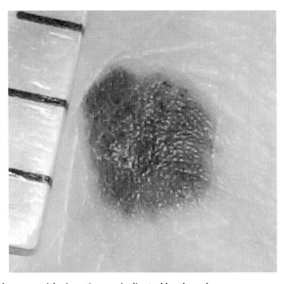

FIGURE 9-17. Melanoma with size >1cm as indicated by the ruler.

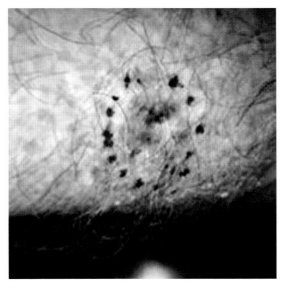

FIGURE 9-18. Amelanotic melanoma.

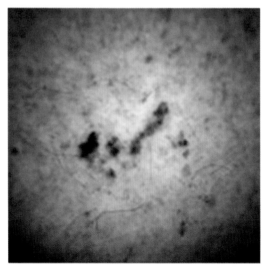

FIGURE 9-19. Melanoma with asymmetric borders.

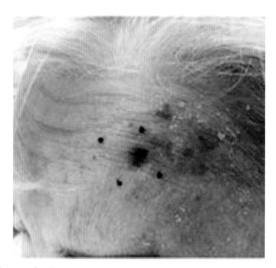

FIGURE 9-20. Melanoma lentigo.

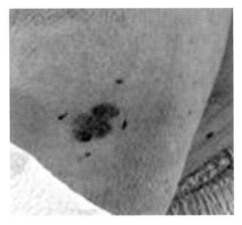

FIGURE 9-21. Invasive melanoma.

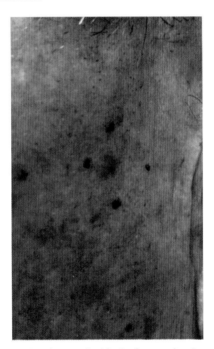

FIGURE 9-22. Collision or junctional nevus (inside the four markers).

Clinical presentation
- Best described by the ABCDE presentation
  - **A**symmetry of the discolored area
  - **B**orders that are uneven and distinct
  - **C**olor that is dark brown or black (Amelanotic melanomas can defy this characteristic)
  - **D**iameter more than 1 cm
  - **E**volution to a larger, darker lesion
- Is classified by depth according to the Breslow and Clark Depth Scales (Table 9-1)

TABLE 9-1.   Breslow and clark depth scales for melanoma

Stage	Depth (Breslow)	Description of Tissue Involvement (Clark)
I	≤ 0.75 mm	Confined to epidermis (in situ)
II	0.75 mm–1.5 mm	Invasion into papillary dermis
III	1.51 mm–2.25 mm	Fills papillary dermis and compresses the reticular dermis
IV	2.25 mm–3.0 mm	Invasion of reticular dermis (localized)
V	>3.0 mm	Invasion of subcutaneous tissue (regionalized by direct extension)

Medical management
- The following tests for diagnosis and prognosis
  - First line is a surgical or shave biopsy to at least the dermal layer—essential to obtain the entire area of concern if possible because partial biopsies may yield false-negative results
  - Pigmented Lesion Assay (PLA)—a non-invasive method that uses an adhesive patch to obtain mRNA from the surface of a suspected melanoma, in lieu of a biopsy[16]
  - myPath Melanoma—a diagnostic test that measures the expression of 23 genes in a suspicious lesion to distinguish a malignant melanoma from a benign nevus
  - DecisionDx-Melanoma test—a gene profile test to help determine recurrence or metastasis of melanoma[17]
  - Genetic testing for patients with a strong familial history of melanoma
- Wide local excision, followed by sentinel node biopsy, hemotherapy, and radiation if needed (refer to current NCCN Guidelines)
- Mohs surgery with immunohistochemistry or slow Mohs for melanoma in situ, thin melanomas, and lentigo maligna

Wound management
- No wound management is indicated unless the excision results in a non-healing wound

MERKEL CELL CARCINOMA (MCC)

Figures 9-23 through 9-28

Pathophysiology
- Is a locally invasive, highly metastatic neuroendocrine skin cancer
- Originates from round Merkel cells located at the basal layer of the epidermis
- Understood to be most commonly triggered by the Merkel cell polyomavirus (MCV), in which the MCV integrates into the malignant genome, resulting in the loss of replicative competence and expression of T cell antigens;[18,19] or by somatic mutations from ultraviolet light[20]
- Has a poorer prognosis if the tumor is virus-negative[21]

- Has the following risk factors:
  - Exposure to ultraviolet radiation
  - Immunosuppression (e.g. AIDS, organ transplant history and anti-rejection medications)
  - Advanced age

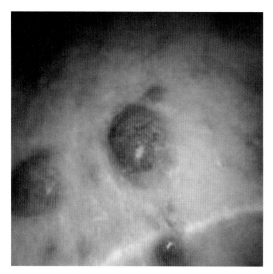

FIGURE 9-23. **Early-stage MCC.**

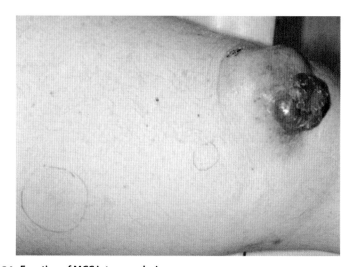

FIGURE 9-24. **Eruption of MCC into open lesion.**

Reproduced with permission from Kang S, Amagai M, Bruckner AL, et al: Fitzpatrick's Dermatology, 9th ed. New York, NY: McGraw Hill; 2019.

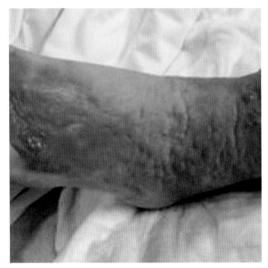

FIGURE 9-25. MCC on the foot and lower leg.

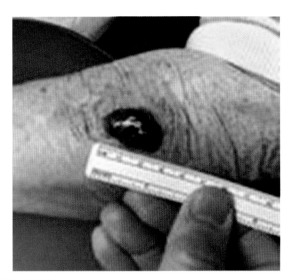

FIGURE 9-26. MCC on the forearm.

Clinical presentation
- Often begins as a painless, firm, solitary, red or violaceous colored, small dermal nodule with a shiny surface and telangiectasias (defined as dilated or wiry small red vessels), usually <2 cm, that rapidly progresses to a larger, ulcerated skin lesion[22]
- Can present as multiple scattered nodules in advanced cases
- May cause lymphedema or pseudo-cellulitis
- Presents most frequently on the face and neck, then the extremities and trunk

Medical management
- Emergent histological diagnosis and baseline staging[23]
- Sentinel lymph node biopsy
- Excision with wider margins (>2 cm)[18]
- Adjuvant radiotherapy and chemotherapy
- Immunotherapy with programmed cell death for late-stage disease[24]

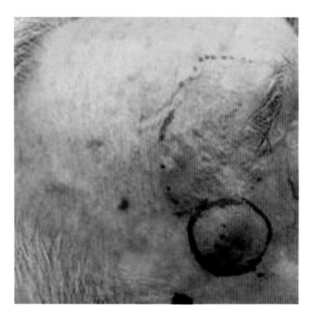

FIGURE 9-27. MCC on the forehead.

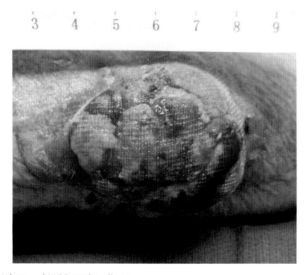

FIGURE 9-28. Advanced MCC on the elbow.

Wound management
- Absorbent antimicrobial dressings on open lesions prior to surgical excision
- No wound management indicated after surgery if the incision heals without complications
- Moist wound therapy if the surgical incision dehisces

KAPOSI SARCOMA

Figures 9-29 through 9-36

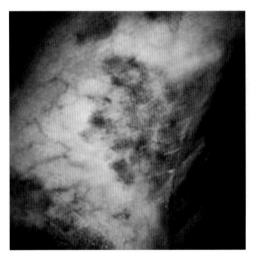

FIGURE 9-29. Kaposi sarcoma.

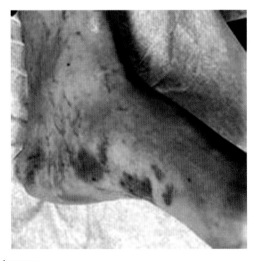

FIGURE 9-30. Kaposi sarcoma.

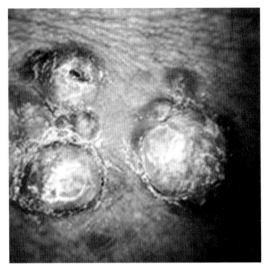

FIGURE 9-31. Kaposi sarcoma.

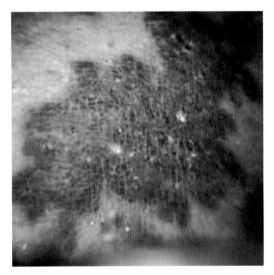

FIGURE 9-32. Kaposi sarcoma.

Pathophysiology
- Is a "multicentric neoplasm of lymphatic endothelium-derived cells infected with Kaposi's sarcoma-associated herpesvirus (KSHV) otherwise called human herpesvirus-8 (HHV-8)"[25]
- Has four clinical subsets:
  - Classic or sporadic—observed most frequently in Mediterranean countries; must have previous infection with HHV-8; has slow progression; predominantly on the extremities

- ○ Endemic—observed in sub-Saharan Africans; predominantly on the extremities
- ○ Iatrogenic—observed in patients treated with immunosuppressive therapy, e.g. after organ transplant; risk peaks in first 2 years after transplant with mean onset at 13 months
- ○ Epidemic—occurs in patients who are HIV-positive[25]
- Occurs in patients infected with HHV-8
- Progression determined by patient's level of immunosuppression
- May occur in internal organs (respiratory system and gastrointestinal tract[26]) without cutaneous lesions[27]

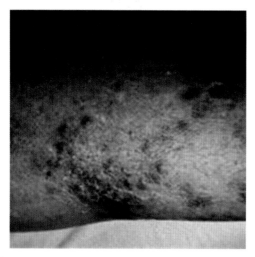

FIGURE 9-33. **Kaposi sarcoma.**

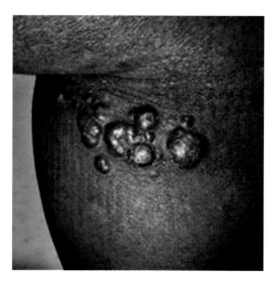

FIGURE 9-34. **Kaposi sarcoma on dark skin.**

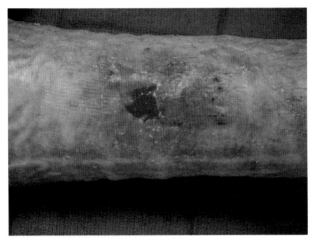

FIGURE 9-35. Traumatic wound on a lower extremity site years after the patient was treated with radiation for Kaposi sarcoma.

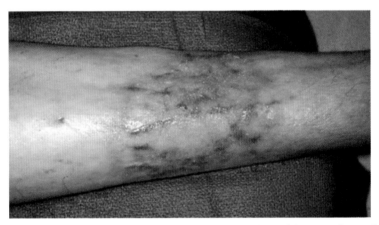

FIGURE 9-36. Healed traumatic wound after treatment with biological dressing, electrical stimulation, and hair follicle transplants.

Clinical presentation
- Presents with purplish, reddish-blue, or dark brown macules, plaques, or nodules
- May bleed and ulcerate
- Is often painless, without notable symptoms, and gradually spreads over time
- Commonly occurs on lower extremities, trunk, or oral cavity,[26] but may occur anywhere including genitals
- Frequently causes lymphedema when on the lower extremities

Medical management
- Confirm diagnosis with biopsy
- Treat localized lesions with the following: alitretinoin gel, aggressive cryotherapy, laser therapy, radiotherapy, or intralesional chemotherapy (paclitaxel,vinblastine, vincristine)[28]

- Avoid surgical excision; associated with high recurrence rate
- Administer systemic treatment if disease is extensive; antiretroviral drugs for HIV-related KS
- Taper immunosuppressive therapy for post-transplant HIV in combination with systemic therapy
- Monitor for recurrence, and educate patient on care of irradiated skin

> **Clinical Guideline:** Procedural and topical treatments of KS are associated with higher recurrence due to the nature of disease pathophysiology.

Wound management
- Topical application of 9-*cis*-retinoic acid (alitretinoin gel) to skin lesions[29]
- Compression therapy for lower extremity edema
- Standard moist wound therapy with adjunctive electrical stimulation and/or HBOT for traumatic wounds that occur on irradiated tissue[30]
- Hair follicle transplants with stem cells to clean granulated lesions that do not respond to standard care

CUTANEOUS LYMPHOMA

*Figures 9-37 **through** 9-40*

Pathophysiology
- Is a heterogeneous group of non-Hodgkin lymphomas that manifest as skin lesions, with or without subsequent extra-cutaneous involvement of the nodes, viscera, and/or blood[31]
- Is classified into T cell and B-cell lymphoma (Table 9-2)
- Involves clonal proliferation of neoplastic T cells or B cells that migrate to the skin and cause lesions

Clinical presentation
- T cell lymphomas (Mycosis fungoides and Sezary syndrome)
  - Present as patches, plaques, or tumors
  - Are flat patches that are scaly or have textural changes *or* plaques with slightly raised lesions that can be smooth, scaly, crusted, or ulcerated
  - Are usually erythematous on presentation, can be hyperpigmented
  - Is termed erythroderma if the presentation is diffuse scaling or confluence of lesions and covers ≥ 80% of the body surface area
  - Presentations specific to mycosis fungoides
    - Poikiloderma
    - Hypopigmented macules and patches
    - Follicular plugging
    - Alopecia
    - Keratoderma
    - Blisters
    - Redundant skin in the axillary or inguinal folds[31]
- B-cell lymphomas
  - Presents with infiltrated plaques, red-to-purple nodules, or tumors (defined as a lesion at least 1 cm in diameter that has vertical growth or depth)[31,32,]

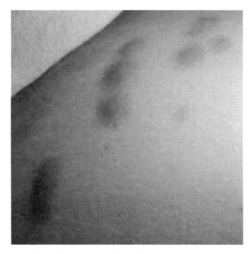

FIGURE 9-37. Early presentation of cutaneous lymphoma.

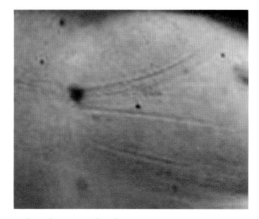

FIGURE 9-38. Cutaneous lymphoma on the chest.

Medical management
- Skin biopsy (incisional, excisional, or punch) for specific diagnosis of lymphoma type, taken at least 2 weeks after any topical steroids or immunosuppressive agents are discontinued[33]
- Examination of skin and lymph nodes, blood work, and CT scans to determine staging
- Chest radiograph to screen for visceral disease
- Skin-directed therapies for first-line treatment (mycosis fungoides and Sezary syndrome)
  - Topical corticosteroids
  - Topical chemotherapeutic agents
  - Topical and systemic retinoids

- o Methotrexate
- o Narrowband UV-B or psoralen-UV-A for early-stage mycosis fungoides[34]
- Polychemotherapy, radiation therapy, extracorporeal photopheresis, and allogenic hematopoietic stem cell transplant for advanced stage disease[33,35,36]

Wound management
- Non-adherent primary dressings and absorbent secondary dressings on open lesions
- Skin moisturizers for pruritis[37]

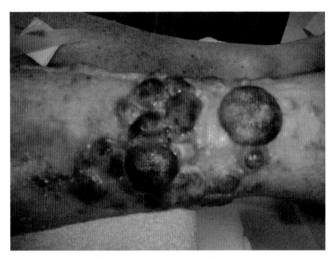

FIGURE 9-39. Advanced mycosis fungoides, a type of T cell lymphoma.

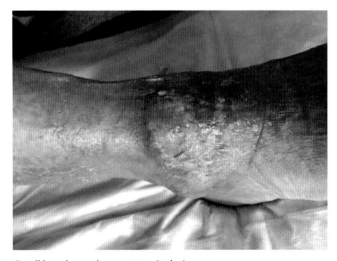

FIGURE 9-40. B-cell lymphoma, lower extremity lesions.

TABLE 9-2.   Classification of primary cutaneous lymphoma (WHO-EORTC)

Cutaneous T Cell and NK Cell Lymphomas
• Mycosis fungoides
• Mycosis fungoides variants and subtypes
• Folliculotropic mycosis fungoides
• Pagetoid reticulosis
• Granulomatous slack skin
• Sézary syndrome
• Adult T cell leukemia/lymphoma
• Primary cutaneous CD30-positive lymphoproliferative disorders
• Primary cutaneous anaplastic large-cell lymphoma
• Lymphomatoid papulosis
• Subcutaneous panniculitis-like T cell lymphoma
• Extranodal NK/T cell lymphoma, nasal type
• Primary cutaneous peripheral T cell lymphoma, unspecified
• Primary cutaneous aggressive epidermotropic CD8$^+$ T cell lymphoma (provisional)
• Cutaneous γ/δ T cell lymphoma (provisional)
• Primary cutaneous CD4$^+$ small- or medium-sized pleomorphic T cell lymphoma (provisional)
Cutaneous B cell lymphomas
• Primary cutaneous marginal zone B cell lymphoma
• Primary cutaneous follicle center lymphoma
• Primary cutaneous diffuse large B cell lymphoma, leg type
• Primary cutaneous diffuse large B cell lymphoma, other
• Intravascular large B cell lymphoma (provisional)
• Precursor hematologic neoplasm
• CD4$^+$/CD56$^+$ hematodermic neoplasm (blastic NK cell lymphoma)

Reproduced with permission from Kang S, Amagai M, Bruckner AL, et al: Fitzpatrick's Dermatology, 9th ed. New York, NY: McGraw Hill; 2019.

PALLIATIVE CARE

Figures 9-41 **through** *9-47*

After tumor removal, patients will sometimes have non-healing wounds or extensive surgical excisions that require palliative care. The treatment goals are not full closure and remodeling, rather they are to minimize pain, to optimize patient function, to eliminate odor, and to allow the patient to have quality time with loved ones.[38] For fungating wounds, often with odiferous drainage, dressings that may help reduce odor include topical metronidazole, Mesalt® (Molnlycke Health Care, Norcross, GA), activated carbon dressing, and curcumin ointment.[39] Hemostatic agents and absorbent alginate dressings may be helpful in stemming the bleeding and drainage that often occur with these wounds (Figure 9-41). Secondary dressings need to be absorbent enough to hopefully allow for less than daily dressing changes. For wounds with copious drainage, silicone-backed thin wicking foams allow the drainage to be absorbed by the outer dressings; the outer dressings can then be changed as needed without disrupting the wound bed (Figures 9-42 and 9-43). This type of dressing can

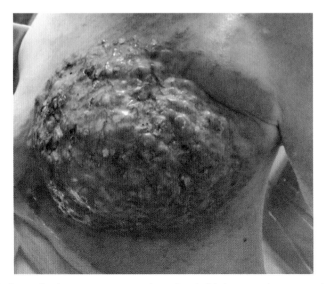

FIGURE 9-41. Fungating breast cancer wound; an absorbable hemostatic agent and silver alginate dressings were used to minimize bleeding and manage exudate.

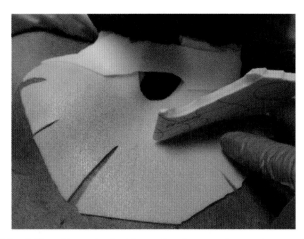

FIGURE 9-42. Thin wicking silicone-backed foam placed over and around a wound after surgery and radiation for a malignant tumor. This layer can be left in place for more than one dressing change.

also allow for family or care-givers to change the secondary dressings without having to visualize the underlying wound. For larger post-surgical wounds, negative pressure wound therapy may be useful although the modality is generally contraindicated for malignant wounds (Figure 9-44).

An integral part of treating a wound caused by surgical removal of a malignant lesion is routine evaluation for recurrence of the tumor at the time of every dressing change (Figures 9-45 and 9-46). The malignant tissue will have some of the characteristics listed in the introduction, as opposed to normal healthy granulation tissue.

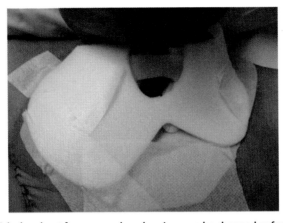

FIGURE 9-43. Thick absorbent foam secondary dressings can be changed as frequently as needed without disturbing the wound bed or causing pain to the patient.

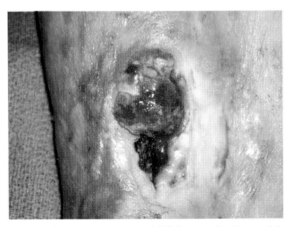

FIGURE 9-44. Negative pressure wound therapy on a large dorsal wound after I&D of a malignant tumor, for a patient on palliative care.

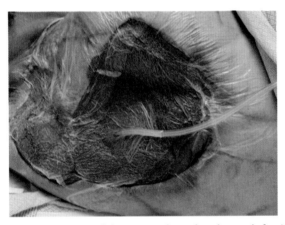

FIGURE 9-45. Recurrence of soft tissue sarcoma visible in a non-healing excisional wound.

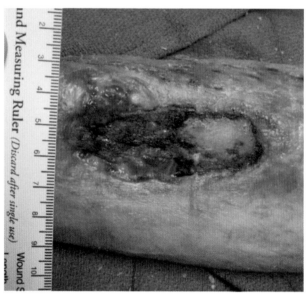

FIGURE 9-46. Recurrence of sarcoma at the tibia edges that are necrotic as a result of radiation.

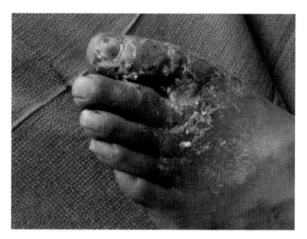

FIGURE 9-47. Hemangioma on the great toe of an adolescent; although present since birth, the character of the lesion changed as a result of becoming a malignancy that required the patient to have a below-knee amputation.

In summary, any wound that does not look normal, is probably not normal and needs further tests to rule out or confirm a diagnosis. An example is the wound in Figure 9-47 that has some characteristics of an ischemic wound; however, the foot is obviously that of a younger individual who in fact had a history of hemangioma on the great toe. The patient history, age, abnormal tissue, and musky odor indicated this may be a malignancy, which indeed it was. Any wound that raises these types of red flags warrants a tissue biopsy in order to make an accurate diagnosis, and thereby initiate appropriate treatment as soon as possible.

REFERENCES

1. Day D, Chakari W, Matzen SH. Malignant transformation of a non-healing wound on the lower extremity: A case report. *Int J Surg Case Reports*. 2018;53:468–470.
2. Maida V, Ennis M, Kuziemsky C, Trozzolo L. Symptoms associated with malignant wounds: A prospective case series. *J Pain & Symptom Management*. 2009;37(2): 206–211.
3. Kyrgidis A, Tzellos TG, Vahtsevanos K, Triadidis S. New concepts for basal cell carcinoma. Demographic, clinical, histological risk factors, and biomarkers: A systematic review of evidence regarding risk for tumor development, susceptibility for second primary and recurrence. *J Surg Res*. 2010;159(1):545-556.
4. Basal cell carcinoma. Available at https://www.mayoclinic.org/diseases-conditions/basal-cell-carcinoma/symptoms-causes/syc-20354187. Accessed April 26, 2020.
5. Firnhaber JM. Diagnosis and treatment of basal cell and squamous cell carcinoma. *Am Fam Physician*. 2012;86(2):161-168.
6. Basal Cell carcinoma. Available at https://en.wikipedia.org/wiki/Basal-cell_carcinoma. Accessed April 27, 2020.
7. Williams HC, Bath-Hextall F, Ozolins M, Armstrong S, Colver GB, Perkins W, et al. Surgery versus 5% imiquimod for nodular and superficial basal cell carcinoma: 5 year results of the SINS random control trial. *J Investigative Dermat*. 2017;137(3):614-619.
8. Jansen MHE, Mosterd K, Arits A, et al. Five-year results of a randomized controlled trial comparing effectiveness of photodynamic therapy, topical imiquimod, and topical 5-fluorouracil in patients with superficial basal cell carcinoma. *J Invest Dermatol*. 2018;138(3):527-533.
9. Glen P, Farrugia D, Farrier J. Complete remission of advanced, locally invasive basal cell carcinoma with vismodegib (Erivedge, Roche Pharmaceuticals). *Head and Neck Oncology*. Available at https://doi.org/10.1016/j.ijom.2020.03.006. Accessed April 24, 2020.
10. Franco R. Basal and squamous cell carcinoma associated with chronic venous leg ulcer. *Intern J Dermatol*. 2001;40:539-544.
11. Kirsner RS, Spencer J, Falanga V, Garland LE, Kerdel FA. Squamous cell carcinoma arising in osteomyelitis and chronic wounds. *Dermatol Surg*. 1996;22(12):1015–1028.
12. Tobin C, Sanger JR. Marjolin's ulcers: a case series and literature review. *Wounds*. 2014;26(9):248-254.
13. Xiong DD, Beal BT, Varra V, Rodriguez M, Cundall H, Woody NM, et al. Outcomes in intermediate-risk squamous cell carcinomas treated with Mohs micrographic surgery compared with wide local excision. *J Am Acad Dermatol*. 2020;82(5):1195-1204.
14. Mabeta P. Paradigms of vascularization in melanoma: Clinical significance and potential for therapeutic targeting. *Biomedicine & Pharmacology*. 2020;127. Available at https://doi.org/10.1016/j.biopha.2020.110135.
15. Wickremesekera HD, Brasch VM, Lee PF, Davis K, Woon K, Johnson R, et al. Expression of cancer stem cell markers in metastatic melanoma to the brain. *J Clin Neurosci*. 2019;60:112-116.
16. Ferris LK, Rigel DS, Siegal DM, Skelsey MK, Peck GL, Hren C, et al. Impact on clinical practice of a non-invasive gene expression melanoma rule-out test: 12-month follow-up

of negative test results and utility data from a large US registry study. *Dermatol Online J.* 2019;25:5. Pii:13030/qt61w6h7mn. Accessed April 29, 2020.

17. Fried BS, Tan A, Bajaj S, Liebman TN, Polsky D, Stein JA. Technological advances for the detection of melanoma: Part II. Advances in molecular techniques. *J Am Acad Dermtol.* 2020. Available at https://doi.org/10.1016/j.jaad.2020.03.122. Accessed April 29, 2020.

18. Steven N, Lawton P, Poulsen. Merkel cell carcinoma – current controversies and future directions. *Clinical Oncology.* 2019;31:789-796.

19. Arora R, Rekhi B, Chandrani P, Krishna S, Dutt A. Merkel cell polyomavirus is implicated in a subset of Merkel cell carcinomas, in the Indian subcontinent. *Microbial Pathogenesis.* 2019;137:103778. Available at https://doi.org/10.1016/j.micpath.2019.103778.

20. Cornejo C, Miller CJ. Merkel cell carcinoma: Updates on staging and management. *Dermatol Clinic.* 2019;37:269-277.

21. Moshiri AS, Doumani R, Yelistratova L, Blom A, Lachance K, Shinohara MM, et al. Polyomavirus-negative Merkel cell carcinoma: A more aggressive subtype based on analysis of 282 cases using multimodal tumor virus detection. *J Invest Dermatol.* 2017; 123(8):1464-1474.

22. Culcu S, Eroglu A, Heper A. Merkel cell carcinoma with axillary metastasis: A case report of a rare disease. *J Oncolog Sci.* 2018;4:53-55.

23. Harms KL, Healy MA, Nghiem P, Sober AJ, Johnson TM, Bichakjian CK, et al. Analysis of prognostic factors from 9387 Merkel cell carcinoma cases forms the basis for the new 8th edition AJCC staging system. *Ann Surg Oncol.* 2016;3(11):3564-3571.

24. Emge DA, Cardones AR. Updates on Merkel cell carcinoma. *Dermatol Clin.* 2019;37:489-503.

25. Lebbe C, Garbe C, Stratigos AJ, Harwood C, Peris K, del Marmol V, et al. Diagnosis and treatment of Kaposi's sarcoma: European consensus-based interdisciplinary guideline (EDF/EADO/EORTC). *Eu J Cancer.* 2019;114:117-127.

26. Caro-Vargas CC, Sellers S, Host KM, Seltzer J, Landis J, Fischer WA, et al. Runaway Kaposi sarcoma-associated herpesvirus replication correlates with systemic IL-10 levels. *Virology.* 2020;539:18-25.

27. Kawakami N, Nmkoong H, Shimoda M, Kotani H, Fujiwara H, Hasegawa N. Hidden disseminated extracutaneous AIDS-related Kaposi sarcoma. *ID Cases.* 2020. Available at https://doi.org/10.1016/j.idcr.2020.e00716. Accessed May 1, 2020.

28. Krown SE, Moser CB, MacPhail P, Matining RM, Godfrey C, Caruso SR, et al. Treatment of advanced AID-associated Kaposi sarcoma in resource-limited settings: A three-arm, open-label, randomized, non-inferiority trial. *Lancet.* 2020;395(4):1195-1207.

29. Gill K, Shah JB. Kaposi sarcoma in patients with diabetes and wounds. *Advances in Skin and Wound Care.* 2006;19(4):196-201.

30. Hamm R, Shah JB. Atypical Wounds. In Hamm R (Ed). *Text & Atlas of Wound Diagnosis and Treatment.* New York: McGraw Hill Education. 2019;235-268.

31. Olsen EA. Evaluatin, diagnosis, and staging of cutaneous lymphoma. *Dermatol Clin.* 2015;33:643-654.

32. Graham PM, Richardson AS, Schapiro BL, Saunders MD, Stewart DM. Spontaneous regression of primary cutaneous diffuse large B-cell lymphoma, leg type with significant T-cell immune response. Available at https://doi.org/10.1016/j.jdcr.2017.10.012.

33. Malachowski SJ, Sun J, Chen P, Seminario-Vidal L. Diagnosis and management of cutaneous B-cell lymphomas. *Dermatol Clin.* 2019;37(4):443-454.

34. Phan K, Ramachandran V, Fassihi H, Sebaratnam DF. Comparison of narrowband UV-B with Psoralen-UV-A phototherapy for patients with early-stage mycosis fungoides: A systematic review and meta-analysis. *JAMA Dermatol.* 2019;155(3):335-341.

35. Iqbal M, Reljic T, Ayala E, Sher T, Murthy H, Roy V, et al. Efficacy of allogeneic hemato-poietic cell transplantation in cutaneous T-cell lymphomaL Results of a systematic review and meta-analysis. *Biol Blood Marrow Transplant.* 2020;26(1):76-82.

36. King B, Lester SC, Tolkachjov SN, Davis M, Gibson LE, Martenson JA. Skin-directed radiation therapy for cutaneous lymphoma: The Mayo Clinic experience. *J Am Acad Dermatol.* 2020;82(3):634-641.

37. Serrano L, Martinez-Escala ME, Xiaolong AZ, Guitart J. Pruritus in cutaneous T-cell lym-phoma and its management. *Dermatol Clin.* 2018;36:245-258.

38. Tilley C, Lipson J, Ramos M. Palliative wound care for malignant fungating wounds. *Nurs Clin N Am.* 2016;51:513-531.

39. Santos C, Pimenta C, Nobre M. A systematic review of topical treatment to control the odor of malignant fungating wounds. *J Pain & Symptom Management.* 2010;39(6):1065-1076.

10

Miscellaneous Wounds

INTRODUCTION

Many wounds, despite their relation to the many pathophysiological processes defined in this handbook, defy simple description. Thus, the miscellaneous wounds discussed in this chapter may have some underlying tendencies of other diagnoses, e.g. an immune component, but have a different unique primary etiology, or even unknown pathophysiology. Because of their unique pathological manifestations, often multi-disciplinary approaches will be required to both diagnose and treat the patient and the wound. Elusive and challenging pathways to both wound healing and subsequent return to optimal function are the only common factors in this group of wounds.

CALCIPHYLAXIS

Figures 10-1 and 10-2

Pathophysiology
- Is caused by calcific occlusion of the small vessels to the skin and subcutaneous tissue
- Is classified as calcific uremic arteriolopathy (CUA) or non-uremic calciphylaxis (NUC)[1] with the risk factors shown in Table 10-1.

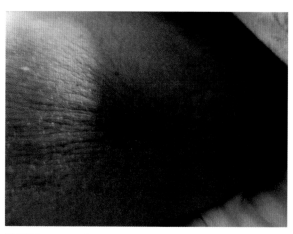

FIGURE 10-1. Early presentation of calciphylaxis.

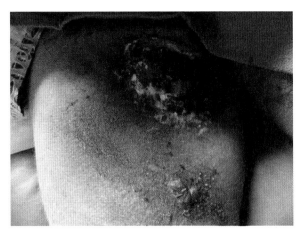

FIGURE 10-2. Progression of calciphylaxis to full thickness, necrotic wounds.

TABLE 10-1.   Risk factors for calcifylaxis

• End-stage renal disease
  • Peritoneal dialysis more than hemodialysis
  • Dialysis more than renal transplant

• Derangements in calcium and phosphate homeostasis
  • Hyperphosphatemia
  • Hypercalcemia
  • Hyper- and hypoparathyroidism
  • Vitamin D

• Vitamin K deficiency associated with warfarin therapy

• Co-morbid conditions
  • Diabetes
  • Obesity
  • Rapid weight loss

• Demographic factors   • Female sex

Adapted from Chang JJ. Calciphylaxis: Diagnosis, pathogenesis, and treatment. Advances in Skin & Wound Care. 2019;32(5):205-215.

- Is not well understood, but CUA appears to be related to deficiencies in vascular calcification inhibitors (e.g. fetuin-A and matrix Gla protein) and dysregulation of extra-skeletal mineralization[1]
- Has the following three-step progression
  - Calcification within the media layer of the vessel causing narrowing of the lumen
  - Proliferation of endothelial cells and fibrosis underneath the intima (termed subintimal fibroplasia)
  - Thrombosis of the vessel lumen resulting in ischemic injury to the skin and hypodermis[2]

Clinical presentation
- Presents initially as livedo reticularis, plaques, or nodules
- Progresses to skin and subcutaneous necrosis with dark eschar
- Causes erythema, induration, and severe pain
- Usually occurs on bilateral lower extremities (especially thighs) and abdomen, areas where there is more adipose tissue
- May occur in areas where patient gives daily insulin injections, due to the repeated trauma[2]

Medical management
- Confirm diagnosis with a punch biopsy using the double trephine technique[2]
- Treat to halt the vascular calcification[2]
  - Increase phosphate removal and decrease phosphate intake (ideal phosphate level is 3 mg/dL)
  - Increase calcium removal by dialysis and decrease calcium intake (ideal calcium level is 8 mg/dL)
  - Lower levels of parathyroid hormone with cinacalcet (in mild cases) or parathyroidectomy in refractory cases[3]
  - Discontinue Vitamin D supplements[4]
  - Discontinue warfarin and substitute alternative anticoagulants[5]
  - Transition from peritoneal dialysis to hemodialysis if possible
  - Administer IV SNF472, 9 mg kg^{-1} to patients on hemodialysis[6,7]
- Decalcify vessels in order to restore blood flow to the tissue[2]
  - Administer sodium thiosulfate through hemodialysis[3,8] and/or by direct injection into the border and center of the lesions,[9] or through negative pressure wound therapy with instillation.[10]
  - Administer oral Vitamin K, now in clinical trials[11]
- Monitor calorie and protein intake to optimize nutritional levels necessary for wound healing[12]
- Manage pain with Fentanyl and methadone (medications which contain no active metabolites that accumulate in renal failure); avoid morphine which has active metabolites and also depresses respiration
- Decrease opioid use as pain diminishes in order to increase alertness, allow participation in rehabilitation, and improve oral intake
- Antibiotics if needed for infection

Wound management
- Meticulous wound care with aseptic technique to prevent infection
- Debridement of all necrotic tissue, either by sharp or surgical technique, depending on the pain levels and amount of tissue to be removed
- Moist wound dressings or negative pressure wound therapy, depending on size of wounds after debridement
- Hyperbaric oxygen therapy to increase tissue perfusion and stimulate granulation
- Split-thickness skin grafts when wounds are clean and fully granulated

WARFARIN-INDUCED SKIN NECROSIS (WISN)

Figures 10-3 and 10-4

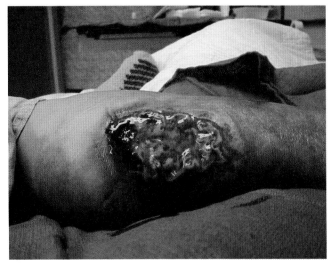

FIGURE 10-3. Warfarin-induced skin necrosis after partial debridement of the necrotic tissue.

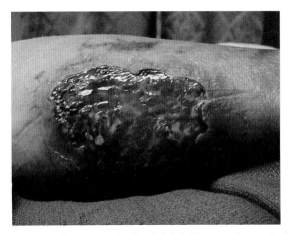

FIGURE 10-4. Warfarin-induced skin necrosis after full debridement of necrotic skin and subcutaneous tissue.

Pathophysiology
- Is also referred to as Coumadin-induced skin necrosis
- Is a rare complication of anticoagulation therapy, usually with warfarin and less frequently with heparin
- Occurs within the first 10 days of initiation of warfarin, although it has been reported to occur with re-initiation of anticoagulation after a break in therapy[13]
- Is often associated with a large initial loading dose of warfarin without simultaneous initial use of heparin[14,15]
- Involves the inactivation of vitamin K-dependent clotting factors, protein C, and protein S which creates a hypercoagulable state[14]

- Presents with diffuse dermal microthrombi with endothelial cell damage and red cell extravasation that together subsequently cause dermal ischemia[17]
- Involves the following risk factors:
  - Deficiency of protein C
  - Deficiency of protein S
  - Factor V Leiden
  - Antithrombin III
  - Hyper-homocysteinaemia
  - Antiphospholipid antibodies
  - Viral infections
  - Hepatic disease[14]

Clinical presentation
- Is more common in middle aged, peri-menopausal, and obese females[15]
- Occurs over areas of the body with adipose, such as the breast, buttocks, thighs, and calves[13]
- Causes initial complaints of paresthesias, pressure sensations, and exquisite pain, followed by edema with *peau d'orange* skin texture[16]
- Presents with painful petechiae that become hemorrhagic lesions and progress rapidly to full-thickness necrosis of the skin and subcutaneous tissue[17]

Medical management
- Immediate discontinuance of the anticoagulant
- Transition to alternate anticoagulant, e.g. IV heparin or dabigatran etexilate
- Vitamin K, protein C concentrates, and prostacyclin for severe cases[14]
- Pain management

Wound management
- Debridement of necrotic tissue by surgical, sharp, or autolytic techniques, depending upon the extent of necrosis and pain levels
- Moist wound therapy with antimicrobial dressings
- Negative pressure wound therapy for larger lesions
- Plastic reconstruction as needed

SICKLE CELL WOUNDS

Figures 10-5 and 10-6

Pathophysiology
- Is a complication of sickle cell disease, a group of hereditary hemolytic anemias characterized by hemoglobin S (HbS) which results in the normal discoid-shaped erythrocyte being shaped like a sickle[18]
- Involves the following processes of abnormal microcirculation and impaired wound healing:
  - Reduced half-life of sickled cells causing hemolytic anemia[18]
  - Abnormal activation of the coagulation cascade and fibrinolysis with increased risk of thrombosis of smaller vessels to the skin[18]
  - Chronic inflammatory state with increased levels of inflammatory markers (e.g. cytokines, chemokines, endothelin-1), chronic hemolysis, ischemia-reperfusion injury, nitric oxide deficiency, and increased numbers of circulating microparticles[18]

- ○ Vaso-occlusion in conjunction with increased adhesion of white blood cells and sickle cells, which causes chronic venous insufficiency and thereby adds to the hypoxia[18]
- ○ Impaired recruitment of endothelial progenitor cells that in turn impairs the cellular proliferation needed for angiogenesis and re-epithelialization, with lower density of both blood and lymph vessels in SC wounds[19]

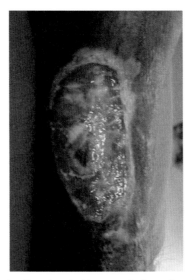

FIGURE 10-5. Non-healing chemical burn on the lower leg of a patient with sickle cell disease.

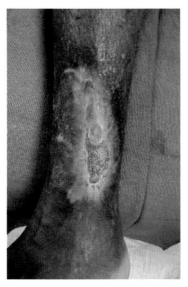

FIGURE 10-6. Sickle cell wound in the proliferative phase of healing.

Clinical presentation
- Occurs in severely anemic SCD patients who are more than 15 years old[19]
- Occurs more frequently in males and individuals who have reduced levels of fetal hemoglobin
- Most commonly occurs spontaneously above the medial malleolus or in a non-healing wound on any area of the lower extremity[20]
- Is exquisitely painful due to the ischemic component
- May present with concomitant chronic venous insufficiency and edema
- Has a shallow wound bed with slough, poor granulation quality, and senescent edges

Medical management
- Blood transfusions to increase oxygen-carrying capacity of blood flow with the goal of keeping hemoglobin levels greater than 10 g/dL[20]
- Administer deferasirox in conjunction with transfusions in order to chelate the excess iron that can accumulate with transfusion[21]
- Hydroxyurea to increase the level of HbF by inhibiting the polymerization of HbS; however, its effect on wound healing has conflicting evidence[20]
- Vascular screening and ankle-brachial index if needed, to determine healing potential of lower extremity wounds
- Pain management
- IV arginine butyrate to help change concentration of abnormal hemoglobin[20,22]
- Pentoxifylline to assist in vasodilation
- Stem cell transplant (through bone marrow transplants from siblings)—a new therapy that will hopefully reduce the complications of SCD, including chronic leg wounds
- Adequate management of lower extremity edema and pre-operative exchange transfusions if patient has skin grafts or other plastic reconstruction[20]
- Physical therapy referral to optimize lower extremity muscle function, range of motion, and cardiac output

Wound management
- Remove necrotic tissue using sharp, autolytic, and enzymatic debridement if the vascular exam shows there is sufficient blood flow for healing; apply topical anesthetic prior to debridement
- Non-contact, low-frequency ultrasound to reduce inflammation and help mitigate pain
- Moist wound healing with dressings to hydrate or absorb exudate as needed
- Antimicrobial dressings if there are signs of critical colonization; systemic antibiotics if there are signs of infection in the surrounding tissue
- Compression therapy to manage edema that is a result of chronic inflammation or chronic venous insufficiency[20]

> **Clinical Guideline:** Dressings that have an anti-inflammatory effect by modulating protease activity include topical collagen, oxidized reduced cellulose (ORC), and silver. For signs of infection in the surrounding tissue, anti-inflammatory antibiotics include doxycycline, cotrimoxazole, clindamydin, and metronidazole.[20]

SPIDER BITES

Figures 10-7 through 10-10

Pathophysiology
- Dermal wounding is usually caused by the brown recluse spider (*Loxosceles reclusa*).
- At the time of the bite, venom is injected into the skin by the hollow modified mouth part called *chelicerae*; counter pressure is required for venom injection when the spider is disturbed.
- The spider is usually found in dark, quiet environments; they are nocturnal and hibernate during the fall, winter, and early spring and only attack when they are disturbed.
- The spiders reside in hot climates and are most prevalent in south-central United States (other species of the brown spider are in other areas, e.g. the Chilean brown spider in South America).[28]

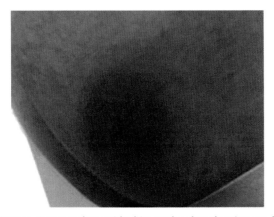

FIGURE 10-7. Brown recluse spider bite on the gluteal region, on day of bite.

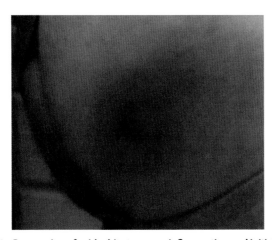

FIGURE 10-8. Progression of spider bite to severe inflammation and initial skin necrosis.

- Tissue necrosis, termed loxoscelism, is the result of a water-soluble substance in the venom that contains eight enzymes (including sphingomyelinase D, hyaluronides, esterase, and alkaline phosphatase).[23]
- Sphingomyelinase D seems to be the most potent component causing the following sequence of tissue injury:
  - Aggregation of platelets with endothelial swelling and destruction
  - Plugging of the capillaries with white cells
  - Ischemia and tissue necrosis[28]

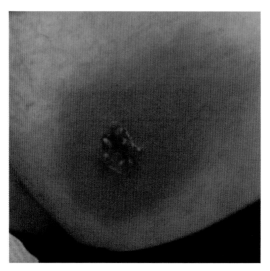

FIGURE 10-9. Spider bite after initial debridement of necrotic tissue.

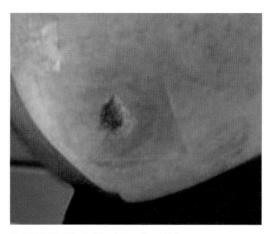

FIGURE 10-10. Spider bite after 17 days.

Clinical presentation
- Initial complaint of stinging or burning sensation
- Immediate formation of a erythematous macule surrounding a central papule[23]; may have two small puncture wounds[27]

- Progression to severe inflammation with a red, white, and blue "bull's eye" appearance in patients who are injected with sufficient venom or who are immune-suppressed
- May become necrotic within 72 hours, with eschar and subcutaneous fatty necrosis
- May develop systemic signs of rash, fever, chills, nausea, vomiting, malaise, arthralgia, and myalgia
- In rare severe cases, may develop renal failure with hemolysis, hemoglobinuria, leukocytosis, leukopenia, or thrombocytopenia[24,25]
- May cause long-term peripheral neuropathy[26]

Medical management
- Cleanse the area well and provide pain relief for immediate care; apply ice pack to prevent spreading of venom (avoid heat); elevate at heart level or higher.[27]
- Administer tetanus toxoid if immunization is not up to date.
- Refer for hyperbaric oxygen therapy if available.[23]
- For systemic symptoms, obtain CBC, chemistry panel, glucose-6-phosphate dehydrogenase (G6PD), and urinalysis; initiate IV fluids to flush kidneys in case of hemolysis, preferably as an in-patient.
- Administer antibiotics to prevent secondary infection.
- May administer dapsone within 24 hours to inhibit neutrophil migration (except in the case of G6PD deficiency).[28]

Wound management
- Debride necrotic tissue when fully demarcated.
- Apply antimicrobial dressings for moist wound healing.
- Refer for plastic reconstruction if not healed after 4–6 weeks.

Diagnostic Clue: Brown recluse spiders and black widow spiders are the two species that have stingers large enough to penetrate the skin. The black widow toxin will cause systemic symptoms, but not dermal wounds. There are four brown recluse species that produce necrotic wounds. Confirmation of the sting etiology is currently only by actual identification of the spider, which the patient is usually unable to provide.[28] A mnemonic to use in differential diagnosis is provided in Table 10-2.

POLYMORPHOUS LIGHT ERUPTION (PMLE)

*Figures 10-11 **through** 10-13*

Pathophysiology
- Is an idiopathic photodermatosis caused by exposure to ultraviolet radiation
- Is the most common photodermatosis, occurring most frequently in temperate climates in early spring and summer, upon first exposure to the sun
- Is thought to be a delayed type IV hypersensitivity response to sunlight-induced cutaneous photoantigens,[29,30] possibly caused by an aberrant reaction of Langerhans cells to ultraviolet exposure[31]

TABLE 10-2.   Mnemonic for differential diagnosis of brown recluse spider bite: NOT RECLUSE

Numerous—the brown recluse spider usually causes only one lesion
Occurrence—usually in a dark place like a closet or attic; only bites when disturbed
Timing—usually between April and October (they hibernate in winter)
Red center—characteristic center of a brown recluse spider bite is pale because of the destruction of the capillary bed
Elevated—if elevated more than 1 cm, it is probably not a brown recluse spider, which is usually flat
Chronic—usually heal within 3 months; if not, consider other issues that may prevent healing or another bite source
Large—brown recluse spider bites are rarely more than 10 cm
Ulcerates too early—usually takes 7–14 days for a brown recluse spider bite to ulcerate
Swollen—may not have significant swelling unless on the foot or face
Exudative—brown recluse spider bites do not typically cause drainage

Data from Stoecker WV, Vetter RS, Dyer JA. NOT RECLUSE-A Mnemonic Device to Avoid False Diagnoses of Brown Recluse Spider Bites, JAMA Dermatol 2017 May 1;153(5):377-378.

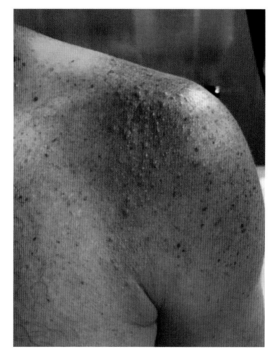

FIGURE 10-11. Polymorphous light eruption.

Clinical presentation
- Development of papules, rash, or eczema on sun-exposed areas not previously exposed, hours to days after exposure to sunlight; may progress to plaques, vesicles, or nodules[29]

- Complaints of pruritus and burning
- Usually resolves spontaneously within 2 weeks, without scarring
- Diminishing severity of outbreak with repeated exposures, termed "hardening"[31]

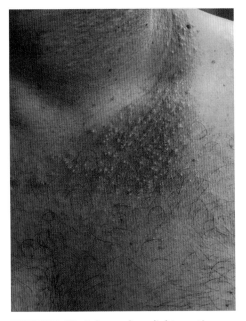

FIGURE 10-12. Polymorphous light eruption.

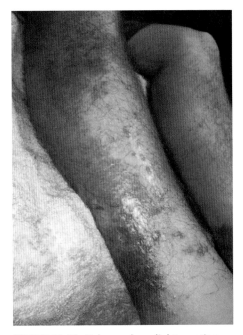

FIGURE 10-13. Polymorphous light eruption.

Medical management
- None indicated unless rare systemic symptoms occur
- Vitamin D replacement if sun is routinely avoided

Wound management
- Prevention
  - Apply a broad-spectrum, water-resistant semi-opaque SPF 50+ sunscreen before sun exposure and every 2 hours thereafter
  - Cover with densely woven clothing when first going out
  - Steadily increase the exposure to sunlight, to induce the "hardening" effect[32]
- Treatment
  - Topical corticosteroids to reduce itching
  - Avoid re-exposure to the sun

FACTITIOUS WOUNDS

Figure 10-14

Pathophysiology
- Is the creation of self-inflicted wounds or the interference with the healing of existing wounds, in order to gain medical attention without any obvious gain[33]
- Is a manifestation of a psychiatric disorder
- Is associated with the warning signs in Table 10-3[34]

Clinical presentation
- Wounds occur on areas of the body that are easy to reach (e.g. face, hands, torso, arms, and legs) and rarely on the back.
- Wounds tend to have geometric edges and healthy granulation tissue.
- *If* dressings are left intact, there will be new wounding at the edges of the dressings.
- Surgical wounds and skin grafts may fail to heal.
- Patients tend to be young, mostly female, and often in some health care profession.[33]

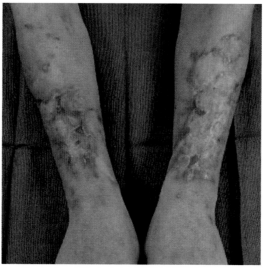

FIGURE 10-14. Factitious wounds on the arms of a physically healthy patient who repeatedly removed dressings and picked at wounds, thus preventing full re-epithelialization.

TABLE 10-3.   Warning signs for patients with factitious wounds

Previous various treatments at multiple hospitals or clinics
Repeated poor outcomes to surgical procedures
Young patient age
Wound in an obvious, easy-to-reach location
Dressings are repeatedly removed between treatment sessions
Wound heals if dressing is left in place
Illness does not follow the natural course of the presumed disease
Patient requests medical procedures or surgery
Patient predicts poor prognosis or deterioration of the wound
Exacerbations occur shortly before or after discharge
Tend to be more educated patients
Demonstrate an angry or hostile profile
Low return-to-work rate
No other explanation for symptoms
Patient resists psychiatric assessment or care

Data from Amr A, Schmitt C, Kuipers T, et al: Identifying and managing patients with factitious wounds, Adv Skin Wound Care 2017 Dec;30(1):1-7 and O'Connor EA, Grunert BK, Matloub HS, et al: Factitious hand disorders: review of 29 years of multidisciplinary care, J Hand Surg Am 2013 Aug;38(8):1590-1598.

Medical management
- Early detection and psychiatric treatment which is critical to successful treatment
- Cognitive behavioral therapy and/or psychodynamic and psychoanalytic therapy, (alone or combined with medication); habit reversal and mentalization-based psychotherapy[35]

Wound management
- Standard moist wound therapy
- Supportive, empathetic care during treatment sessions
- Frequent follow-up treatments

SUMMARY

In summary, this group of miscellaneous wounds is very challenging to every wound care practitioner. Creative application of standard care for wounds of other etiologies is often the basis of treatment, along with addressing the specific underlying circumstances of each unusual case. In addition, patience and persistence by both the practitioner and the patient will facilitate wound healing and in turn allow a return to the prior level of function.

REFERENCES

1. Nigwekar SU, Wolf M, Stems RH, Hix JK. Calciphylaxis from nonuremic causes: A systematic review. *Clin J Am Soc Nephrol.* 2008;3(4):1139-1143.
2. Chang JJ. Calciphylaxis: Diagnosis, pathogenesis, and treatment. *Advances in Skin & Wound Care.* 2019;32(5):205-215.
3. Floege J, Kubo Y, Floege A, Chertow GM, Parfrey PS. The effect of cinacalcet on calcific uremic arteriolopathy events in patients receiving hemodialysis: The EVOLVE Trial. *Clin J Am Soc Nephrol.* 2015;10(5):800-807.
4. Nigweker SU, Zhao DB, Wenger J, et al. A nationally representative study of calcific uremic arteriolopathy risk factors. *J Am Soc Nephrol.* 2016;27:3421-3429.
5. Nigwekar SU, Kroshinsky D, Nazarian RM, et al. Calciphylaxis: Risk factors, diagnosis, and treatment. *Am J Kidney Dis.* 2015;66(1):133-146.
6. Perello J, Joubert PH, Ferrer MD, Canals AZ, Sinha S, Salcedo C. First-time-in-human randomized clinical trial in healthy volunteers and haemodialysis patients with SNF472, a novel inhibitor of vascular calcification. *Br J Clin Pharmacol.* 2018;84(12):2867-2876.
7. Brandenburg VM, Sinha S, Torregrosa JV, Garg R, Miller S, Canals AZ, et al. Improvement in wound healing, pain, and quality of life after 12 weeks of SNF472 treatment: A phase 2 open-label study of patients with calciphylaxis. *J Nephrol.* 2019;32(5):811–821.
8. Peng T, Zhuo L, Wang Y, Jun M, Li G, Wang L, Hong D. Systematic review of sodium thiosulfate in treating calciphylaxis in chronic kidney disease patients. *Nephrology.* 2018;23(7):669-675.
9. Zuhaili B, Al-Talib K. Successful treatment of single infected calciphylaxis lesion with intralesional injection of sodium thiosulfate at high concentration. *Wounds.* 2019;31(8):E54-E57.
10. Herskovitz I, MacQubae FE, Borda LJ, Bhagwandin S, Paredes JA, Polanco T, et al. A novel topical wound therapy delivery system. *Wounds.* 2017;29(9):269-274.
11. Nigwekar SU, Krinsky S, Thadani RI, et al. Phase 2 trial of phytonadione in calciphylaxis. Presented at the American Society of Nephrology's Kidney Week 2019 meeting held Nov. 5 to 10 in Washington, DC. Poster TH-PO1188.
12. Hamm R, Shah JB. Atypical wounds. In Hamm R, ed. *Text & Atlas of Wound Diagnosis and Treatment.* New York, NY: McGraw-Hill Education. 2019;235-268.
13. Lennox AF, Smout J, Shlebak A, Wolfe JHN. Warfarin-induced skin necrosis: Association with heparin-induced thrombocytopenia and protein S deficiency. *Available at https://doi.10.1053/ejvx.2000.0011. Accessed May 7, 2020.*
14. Kakagia KK, Papanas N, Karadimas E, Polychronidis A. Warfarin-induced skin necrosis. *Ann Dermatol.* 2014;26(1):96-98.
15. Roche-Nagle G, Robb W, Ireland A, Bourchier-Hayes D. Extensive skin necrosis associated with warfarin sodium therapy. *Eur J Vasc Endovasc Surg.* 2003;25:481-482.
16. Cheng A, Scheinfeld NS, McDowell B, et al. Warfarin skin necrosis in post-partum woman with protein S deficiency. *Obstet Gynecol.* 1997;90(4, pt 2):671-672.
17. Nazarian RM, Van Cott EM, Zembowicz A, Duncan LM. Warfarin-induced skin necrosis. *J Am Acad Dermatol.* 2009;61(2):325-332.
18. De Toledo SL, Guedes J, Alpoim PN, Rios DRA, de B. Pinheiro M. Sickle cell disease: Hemostatic and inflammatory changes, and their interrelation. *Clinica Chimica Acta.* 2019;493:129-137.
19. Nguyen VT, Nassar D, Batteux F, Raymond K, Tharaux P, Aractingi S. Delayed healing of sickle cell ulcers is due to impaired angiogenesis and CXCL12 secretion in skin wounds. *J Investigative Dermatol.* 2016;136:497-506.
20. Ladizinski B, Bazakas A, Mistry N, Alavi A, Sibbald RG, Salcido R. Sickle cell disease and leg ulcers. *Adv Skin Wound Care.* 2012;25(9):420-428.

21. Hamm RL, Weitz I, Rodrigues J. Pathophysiology and multi-disciplinary management of leg wounds in sickle cell disease: A case discussion and literature review. *Wounds.* 2006;18(10):277-285.

22. Morris C, Kuypers FA, Larkin S, et al. Arginine therapy: A novel strategy to induce nitric oxide production in sickle cell disease. *Br J Haematol.* 2000;111(2):498–500.

23. Haddany A, Fishlev G, Bechor Y, Meir O, Efrati S. Nonhealing wounds caused by brown spider bites: Application of hyperbaric oxygen therapy. *Adv Skin Wound Care.* 2016;29(12):560–566.

24. Suchard JR. "Spider bite" lesions are usually diagnosed as skin and soft-tissue infection. *J Emerg Med.* 2011;41(5):473–481.

25. Isbister GK, White J. Clinical consequences of spider bites: Recent advances in our understanding. *Toxicon.* 2004;43(5):477–492.

26. Delasotta LA, Orozco F, Ong A, Sheikh E. Surgical treatment of a brown recluse spider bite: A case study and literature review. *J Foot & Ankle Surg.* 2014;53(3):320–323.

27. Anoka IA, Robb EL, Baker MB. Brown recluse spider toxicity. 2020, StatPearls Publishing LLC. Available at https://www.ncbi.nlm.nih.gov/books/NBK537045/. Accessed May 10, 2020.

28. Wilson JR, Hagood CO, Prather ID. Brown recluse spider bites: A complex problem wound. A brief review and case study. *Ostomy & Wound Management.* 2005;51(3):59–66.

29. Chen Y, Lee J. Clinicopathologic study of solar dermatitis, a pinpoint papular variant of polymorphour light eruption in Taiwan, and review of the literature. *J of Formosan Med Assn.* 2013;112:125–130.

30. Gruber-Wackernagel A, Byrne SN, Wolf P. Polymorphous light eruption: Clinic aspects and pathogenesis. *Dermatol Clin.* 2014;32:315–334.

31. Kolgen W, Weelden HV, Hengst SD, Guikers K, Kiekens R, Knol EF, et al. CD11b+ cells and ultraviolet-B-resistant CD1a+ cells in skin of patients with polymorphous light eruption. *J Invest Dermatol.* 1999;113(1):4–10.

32. Polymorphous light eruption. Available at https://en.wikipedia.org/wiki/Polymorphous_light_eruption. Accessed May 11, 2020.

33. Yates GP, Feldman MD. Factitious disorder: A systematic review of 455 cases in the professional literature. *General Hospital Psychiatry.* 2016;41:20–28.

34. Amr A, Schmitt C, Kuipers T, Schoeller T, Eckhardt-Henn A, Werdin F. Identifying and managing patients with factitious wounds. *Adv Skin Wound Care.* 2017;30(12):1–7.

35. Tomas-Aragones L, Consoli SM, Consoli SG, Poot F, Taube KM, Linder MD, et al. Self-inflicted lesions in dermatology: A management and therapeutic approach. A position paper from the European Society for Dermatology and Psychiatry. *Acta Derm Venereol.* 2017;97(2):159–172.

Appendix

Identifying Wounds by Anatomical Locations

Index